Disease, Pain, & Sacrifice

WITHDRAWN

When I thought to know this,
it was too painful for me

PSALM 73:16

David Bakan

Disease, Pain, & Sacrifice

Toward a *Psychology of Suffering*

BEACON PRESS

For
Jacob Manuel
and all children
mine and others
Torah, Huppah, u'Maasim Tovim

Preface

Some considerations that aim at augmenting our understanding of human suffering are advanced in this volume. Human understanding and suffering are reflexively related. A certain level of awareness is a precondition for suffering as well as its management; and awareness is enhanced as well as diminished by suffering. Because of these reflexive relationships, oblivion and the enhancement of understanding are two natural options for coping with suffering. I have placed an epigraph facing the title page from the King James translation of the Psalms (which may be more to the credit of the translator than the author). It is not there as a motto to be followed. It is a reminder of one of the most significant mechanisms that interfere with understanding. The thought expressed in the following chapters is informed by the conviction that amelioration of suffering through understanding is the superior option. Temporary or partial oblivion is not without merit. But permanent or complete oblivion is indistinguishable from death. Man, having been endowed with understanding, should cultivate and use it.

Human suffering has biological, psychological, and existential aspects. For the purposes of exposition the first chapter, dealing with disease, stresses the biological aspects; the second, with pain, the psychological aspects;

and the third, using the Book of Job as a springboard, the existential aspects. Tearing asunder and joining is, as will become evident to the reader, the basic theme. I have tried to communicate this also in the form of the book. It is composed of three panels hinged together, a triptych, as it were. Although the biological, psychological, and existential are thus divided, all three are entailed in each of the panels.

Contents

ix

Contents

I

Disease as Telic Decentralization

I am troubled;
I am bowed down greatly;
I go mourning all the day long.
For my loins are filled
with a loathsome disease: and there is no soundness
in my flesh.
PSALM 38:6–7

*H*ow shall human suffering be conceptualized? Disease is certainly one of the most conspicuous manifestations of suffering and thus invites itself as our starting point. The attempt to understand and to manage disease is itself one of man's most ubiquitous characteristics. There has never been a culture which has not concerned itself with disease. Indeed there are few things that are as natural to man as trying to cope with disease, unless it be disease itself.

Disease is central to the total existential condition of mankind. Disease, as death, is inevitable in that eventually death results from a condition which we classify under the rubric of disease. There is much in man's thought, will, temper, art, and science that can determine the occurrence and course of disease. Yet we should not fall into the trap of believing that, since we can do a great deal with respect to the prevention and management of disease, we can prevent death from occurring. In the same way that in religious contexts some have been entrapped into believing that one can achieve personal immortality through devoutness, so can one be tempted into believing in physical immortality by the appearance of great medical achievements in the management of disease. Both are mistaken beliefs, even if it is not mistaken to believe that in some in-

3

stances the quality of religiousness may be associated with longevity, as has been asserted by Sorokin, who found saints to have been especially long-lived,[1] and even if medical measures do lengthen life.

Disease and Separation-Estrangement

There is a growing body of literature which indicates in various ways that the disease process may be dependent upon the equilibrium of the individual in his total life context, especially the social context.

The authors of the Bible considered being "cut off" as the ultimate disaster, source of grief, or punishment that anyone might suffer. Thus, for example, in the story of Job, which I shall deal with at some length later on in this volume, they hardly saw fit completely to separate psychological and physical suffering, the losses of children and property that he suffered and the boils on his body, separation-estrangement and conspicuous physical affliction.

Moore and Anderson have astutely suggested that the contemporary scientific enterprise is quite continuous with the folk culture of ancient times, that both the folk culture and science are basically "models with the help of which we come to understand and 'be at home with' our natural and social environments."[2] As they see the matter, "one of the principal activities of social scientists will be, or should be, to continue the work

---

[1] P. A. Sorokin, *Altruistic love* (Boston: Beacon Press, 1950).

[2] O. K. Moore and A. R. Anderson, "Some puzzling aspects of social interaction," *Review of Metaphysics* 15 (1962): 412.

begun (for our civilization) by Homer and Hesiod; i.e. to continue the job of constructing folk models for the instruction and diversion of our fellow-creatures."[3] Replacing the folk culture with the scientific report is perhaps indicative of progressive enlightenment. Let us, however, reserve the possibility of considering them at least as overlapping categories, instead of conceiving of either the scientific report as a special instance of a folktale or the folktale as a special instance of a scientific report.

For the next few pages I shall take a kaleidoscopic look at scientific reports from the literature. I shall not dwell on any one of them. What is important for our purposes is only that in one way or another each study points to a relationship between what the biblical authors might have referred to as being "cut off" and disease.

The fact that the course of cancer development in animals seems to be related to the "social" condition of their lives should come as a powerful parable for modern man. There is a strain of experimental mouse, designated as C3H, in which mammary cancer develops almost invariably in the female. It has been reported that, among these mice, those raised in cages with cage mates develop cancer substantially, and statistically significantly, later than those raised in cages alone.[4] It has also been found that the time at which cancer symptoms manifest themselves in rats which have been in-

---

[3] *Ibid.*, p. 431.

[4] H. B. Andervont, "Influence of environment on mammary cancer in mice," *Journal of the National Cancer Institute* 4 (1944): 579–81. Skeptical of this finding, we decided to repeat it. This was ably done by my student Barry Dworkin, with the cooperation of Dr. E. Simmons, confirming the Andervont findings.

jected with a cancer-provoking substance is delayed if the rats are handled regularly by humans.[5]

The mortality rate among human infants who are deprived of mothering, even while getting adequate physical care, is substantially greater than among infants not so deprived.[6] Maternal deprivation, described by the investigators as taking "the form of rejection, isolation from social contacts, and neglect; physical abuse and malnutrition . . . occasionally associated," leads to retarded physical growth, delayed maturation of the bones, and retarded psychomotor development in children.[7] The mortality rate for persons in the first year of living in a home for the aged is considerably higher than for comparable aged persons living in their normal home conditions.[8]

Somatic diseases resulting from traumatic disruption of social relations have been demonstrated to occur as quickly as within twenty-four hours.[9] Separation and estrangement from significant persons—actual, anticipated, or symbolic—have been implicated as factors in

[5] G. Newton, "Early experience and resistance to tumour growth," in D. M. Kissen and L. L. LeShan, eds., *Psychosomatic aspects of neoplastic disease* (Philadelphia: J. B. Lippincott, 1964), pp. 71–79.

[6] R. Spitz, *The first year of life* (New York: International Universities Press, 1965).

[7] R. G. Patton and L. I. Gardner, *Growth failure in maternal deprivation* (Springfield, Ill.: Charles C Thomas, 1963), p. 81.

[8] M. A. Lieberman, "Relationship of mortality rates to entrance to a home for the aged," *Geriatrics* 16 (1961): 515–19; D. Miller and M. A. Lieberman, "The relationship of affect state and adaptive capacity to reactions to stress," *Journal of Gerontology* 20 (1965): 492–97.

[9] A. H. Schmale, Jr., "Relationship of separation and depression to disease," *Psychosomatic Medicine* 20 (1958): 259–77.

numerous diseases: asthma,[10] cancer,[11] congestive heart failure,[12] diabetes mellitus,[13] disseminated lupus erythematosus,[14] functional uterine bleeding,[15] Raynaud's dis-

[10] T. M. French, "Psychogenic factors in asthma," *American Journal of Psychiatry* 96 (1939): 87–101.

[11] Elida Evans, *A psychological study of cancer* (New York: Dodd, Mead, 1926); W. A. Greene, Jr., "Psychological factors and reticuloendothelial disease. I. Preliminary observations on a group of males with lymphomas and leukemias," *Psychosomatic Medicine* 16 (1954): 220–30, and "Role of vicarious object in the adaptation to object loss. I. Use of a vicarious object as a means of adjustment to separation from a significant person," *ibid.* 20 (1958): 344–50; W. A. Greene, Jr., L. E. Young, and S. N. Swisher, "Psychological factors and reticuloendothelial disease. II. Observations on a group of women with lymphomas and leukemias," *ibid.* 18 (1956): 284–303; W. A. Greene, Jr., and G. Miller, "Psychological factors and reticuloendothelial disease. IV. Observations on a group of children and adolescents with leukemia: An interpretation of disease development in terms of the mother-child unit," *ibid.* 20 (1958): 124–44; S. J. Kowal, "Emotions as a cause of cancer," *Psychoanalytic Review* 42 (1955): 217–27; L. L. LeShan and R. E. Worthington, "Some psychologic correlates of neoplastic disease: a preliminary report," *Quarterly Review of Psychiatry and Neurology* 16 (1955): 281–88; H. L. Muslin and W. J. Pieper, "Separation experience and cancer of the breast," *Psychosomatics* 3 (1962): 230–36; S. Peller, "Cancer and its relations to pregnancy, to delivery, and to marital and social status. I. Cancer of the breast and genital organs. II. Cancer of organs other than reproductive; total cancer mortality," *Surgery, Gynecology and Obstetrics* 71 (1940): 1–8, 181–86.

[12] W. N. Chambers and M. F. Reiser, "Congestive heart failure," *Psychosomatic Medicine* 15 (1953): 38–60.

[13] L. E. Hinkle, Jr., and S. Wolf, "A summary of experimental evidence relating life stress to diabetes mellitus," *Journal of Mt. Sinai Hospital* 19 (1952): 537–70.

[14] A. R. McClary, E. Meyer, and E. L. Weitzman, "Observations on the role of the mechanism of depression in some patients with disseminated lupus erythematosus," *Psychosomatic Medicine* 17 (1955): 311–21.

[15] M. Heiman, "The role of stress situations and psychological factors in functional uterine bleeding," *Journal of Mt. Sinai Hospital*

ease,[16] rheumatoid arthritis,[17] thyrotoxicosis,[18] tuberculosis,[19] and ulcerative colitis.[20]

Death rates during the first six years after liberation among Americans who had been in prisoner-of-war camps in the Pacific theater in World War II were substantially higher than statistical expectation. These included deaths not only resulting from causes such as tuberculosis, intestinal disorders, and suicide, which

---

23 (1956): 775–81. Dr. Heiman closes his contribution by citing Mark 5:25–34, evidently a preoccupation of one of his female patients. This tells of "a certain woman, which had an issue of blood twelve years" who was cured by touching the garment of Jesus.

[16] J. A. F. Millet, H. Lief, and B. Mittelmann, "Raynaud's disease: psychogenic factors and psychotherapy," *Psychosomatic Medicine* 15 (1953): 61–65.

[17] A. O. Ludwig, "Psychogenic factors in rheumatoid arthritis," *Bulletin of Rheumatic Diseases* 2 (1952): 15–16.

[18] Agnes Conrad, "The psychiatric study of hyperthyroid patients," *Journal of Nervous and Mental Diseases* 79 (1934): 505–29, 656–76; H. J. Kleinschmidt, S. E. Waxenberg, and Ruth Cuker, "Psychophysiology and psychiatric management of thyrotoxicosis: a two year follow-up study," *Journal of Mt. Sinai Hospital* 23 (1956): 131–53; T. Litz, "Emotional factors in the etiology of hyperthyroidism," *Psychosomatic Medicine* 11 (1949): 2–8; B. Mittelmann, "Psychogenic factors and psychotherapy in hyperthyreosis and rapid heart imbalance," *Journal of Nervous and Mental Diseases* 77 (1933): 465–88.

[19] D. M. Kissen, "Specific psychological factors in pulmonary tuberculosis," *Health Bulletin* (issued by the Chief Medical Office of the Department of Health for Scotland) vol. 14 (1956), "The relapse in pulmonary tuberculosis due to specific psychological causes," *ibid.* vol. 15 (1957), and *Emotional factors in pulmonary tuberculosis; an evaluation of psychological factors in onset and relapse and their significance in management, treatment and prevention* (London: Tavistock Publications, 1958); E. Wittkower, *A psychiatrist looks at tuberculosis* (London: National Association for the Prevention of Tuberculosis, 1949).

[20] G. L. Engel, "Studies of ulcerative colitis. III. The nature of the psychologic processes," *American Journal of Medicine* 19 (1955): 231–56.

might be readily understood as residual from the camp experiences, but also deaths from cancer and accidents. Twice the expected number died of cancer, and three times the expected number by accidents.[21]

There is accumulating evidence that the duration of illness among persons is associated with psychological indicants, that the more favorable the indicants with respect to the mental health of the individual, the shorter the duration of the illness.[22] There is evidence also that the psychological condition of patients is a good prognosticator of the effectiveness of medical treatment.[23] The incidence of somatic disease among persons with definite psychological disturbance is substantially greater than normally expected,[24] and a relationship be-

[21] H. G. Wolff, "A concept of disease in man," *Psychosomatic Medicine* 24 (1962): 25–30.

[22] A. Querido, "Forecase and follow-up. An investigation into the clinical, social and mental factors determining the result of hospital treatment," *British Journal of Preventive and Social Medicine* 13 (1959): 33–49; K. Brodman, B. Mittelmann, D. Wechsler, A. Weider, and H. G. Wolff, "The relation of personality disturbances to duration of convalescence from acute respiratory infection" and "The incidence of personality disturbances and their relation to age, rank and duration of hospitalization in patients with medical and surgical disorders in a military hospital," *Psychosomatic Medicine* 9 (1947): 37–44, 45–49; N. S. Greenfield, R. Roessler, and A. P. Crosley, "Ego strength and length of recovery from infectious mononucleosis," *Journal of Nervous and Mental Diseases* 128 (1959): 125–28.

[23] T. H. Holmes, J. R. Joffe, J. W. Ketcham, and T. F. Sheehy, "Experimental study of prognosis," *Journal of Psychosomatic Research* 5 (1961): 235–52; H. S. Abram and B. F. Gill, "Predictions and postoperative psychiatric complications," *New England Journal of Medicine* 265 (1961): 1123–28; Beatrice D. Berle, Ruth H. Pinsky, S. Wolf, and H. G. Wolff, "A clinical guide to prognosis in stress disease," *Journal of the American Medical Association* 149 (1952): 1624–28.

[24] J. W. L. Doust, "Psychiatric aspects of somatic immunity: differential incidence of physical disease in the histories of psychi-

tween psychological disorder and various forms of socio-cultural separation and disintegration has been indicated in a large number of studies.[25]

Some of the observations I have cited obviously raise the question of the sequence of psychological and somatic manifestation of disturbance. In a group of patients with undulant fever (brucellosis) it was found that the amount of time the patients continued to manifest symptoms was greater in those in whom there were indications of depression.[26] In a study of convalescence from influenza, investigators administered the Minnesota Multiphasic Personality Inventory to a group of 600 persons, out of which 26 persons *later* became ill with Asian flu. Of these 26 persons, 14 persons recovered in

---

atric patients," *British Journal of Social Medicine* 6 (1952): 49–67; R. Roessler and N. S. Greenfield, "Incidents of somatic disease in psychiatric patients," *Psychosomatic Medicine* 23 (1961): 413–19.

[25] Alice Balint, "Love for the mother and mother love," trans. M. Balint, *International Journal of Psychoanalysis* 30 (1949): 251–59; Therese F. Benedek, "Toward the biology of the depressive constellation," *Journal of the American Psychoanalytic Association* 4 (1956): 389–427; E. Bibring, "The mechanism of depression," in Phyllis Greenacre, ed., *Affective disorders* (New York: International Universities Press, 1953); W. R. D. Fairbairn, *An object-relations theory of the personality* (New York: Basic Books, 1954); S. Freud, "Mourning and melancholia," in *Collected papers* (London: Hogarth Press, 1946) 4:152–70; E. Jacobson, "Contribution to the metapsychology of cyclothymic depression," in Phyllis Greenacre, ed., *Affective disorders* (New York: International Universities Press, 1953); Melanie Klein, "A contribution to the psychogenesis of manic-depressive states," *Contributions to psychoanalysis, 1921–45* (London: Hogarth Press, 1948); Dorothea C. Leighton, J. S. Harding, D. B. Macklin, A. M. Macmillan, and A. H. Leighton, *The character of danger: psychiatric symptoms in selected communities* (New York: Basic Books, 1963); S. Rado, "The problem of melancholia," *International Journal of Psychoanalysis* 9 (1928): 420–38.

[26] J. B. Imboden, A. Canter, and L. Cluff, "Symptomatic recovery from medical disorders," *Journal of the American Medical Association* 178 (1961): 1182–84.

14 days or less and 12 persons manifested symptoms for 21 days or longer. The mean depressive score on the test, which had been taken 3 to 6 months in advance of the onset of influenza, was significantly and substantially higher for the latter group.[27] Mean scores on the depressive and hypomania scales of the Minnesota Multiphasic Personality Inventory of persons who later develop cardiac disease are significantly higher than normal.[28] Certainly relationships between psychological and physical disorder are not exhaustively explained in terms of the psychological reaction of persons to the actual occurrence of physical illness.

The Doctrine of Specific Etiology of Disease

An obstacle in the way of developing an adequate notion of disease is the so-called *doctrine of specific etiology*, that for every disease there is a specific cause. The doctrine of specific etiology received its major support from the nineteenth century discovery of the role of microscopic organisms in some diseases. In earlier centuries when disease and fatality were so closely linked, there was little problem in distinguishing the well from the sick, with death the proof of pre-existent illness. It was during the nineteenth century that the researches of men like Koch and Pasteur, in identifying bacteria as a cause of disease and finding ways of combating bacterially caused diseases, rendered support to the more

[27] J. B. Imboden, A. Canter, and L. Cluff, "Convalescence from influenza: study of psychological and clinical determinants," *American Medical Association Archives of Internal Medicine* 108 (1961): 393–99.

[28] A. M. Ostfeld, Abstracts of the annual meeting of the American Psychosomatic Society, 1961.

general notion of specificity as a universal characteristic of all diseases. The advances in microscopy fostered the hope, at times indistinguishable from belief, that every alteration in tissue had its specific etiological agent. Our knowledge today, however, even of those diseases that critically involve microscopic organisms, tends to indicate that in most diseases there are several factors; and although that for some diseases there are some *necessary* factors, such as the presence of the tubercle bacillus in tuberculosis, there are other factors associated with the sufficient determination of the disease. Developments in experimental pathology have made us aware that grossly different agents may be evocative of reactions indistinguishable from one another.[29] Some contemporary medical thought has tended to deviate from the doctrine of specific etiology, turning more and more to the consideration of "host" factors, for example, and recognizing the multiplicity of components in disease. As one medical researcher put it a few years ago:

> There is no doubt that the doctrine of specific etiology has constituted an instrument of unmatched power for the experimental study of pathological processes and has been responsible for most of the great advances, theoretical and practical, realized in medicine during the past century.
>
> It is now apparent, however, that the concept of single etiology often fails to provide a complete explanation for the pathogenesis of diseases under natural conditions. . . . In practically all infectious and metabolic disorders, physiological and environ-

[29] See H. G. Wolff, *Stress and disease* (Springfield, Ill.: Charles C Thomas, 1953), p. 3.

mental factors can readily be shown to be important determinants of the disease process.[30]

Some recent evidence suggests that disease may be conceived of as a manifestation of a deeper disorder involving the total condition of the individual and that a specific disease from which any individual appears to be suffering may be regarded as its manifestation.

It is commonplace in psychiatric and psychological practice to distinguish firmly between disorder and symptom, and especially to recognize that the removal of a symptom may hardly be considered a cure of the disorder. The disorder may be expected to manifest itself in some other symptom if only the symptom is removed. Removing symptoms connected with psychological disorders is relatively easy, but responsible clinicians working with such disorders hardly limit themselves to symptoms alone. This insight characteristic of psychiatric and psychological practice—that disorder is not the same as symptom and is more basic than symptom—is equally relevant in many disorders in which the manifestation is primarily somatic. There are some indications of a growing trend among medical practitioners to take cognizance of this possibility.

It may even be true that psychiatry and psychology have benefited by not usually having so easy a way to distinguish between health and sickness as a simple laboratory test of tissue or other matter taken from a patient;[31] that the tendency to make generalizations

[30] R. J. Dubos, "The gold-headed cane in the laboratory," *Public Health Reports* 69 (1954): 366.

[31] For an interesting account of the struggles in connection with definition in the mental health field, see D. Offer and M. Sabshin, *Normality: theoretical and clinical aspects of mental health* (New York: Basic Books, 1966).

about all mental disorders from the one instance where infection plays a definitive role in mental disorder—syphilitic infection in general paresis—has handicapped psychiatry and psychology; and that the Kraepelinian approach, which attempted to classify mental disorders in terms of symptom-complexes that could lead to the specific bodily conditions responsible for each disease, literally held back progress for several decades.

One series of studies is particularly telling in demonstrating the limitations of the doctrine of specific etiology, the investigations by Hinkle and his co-workers.[32] Empirical findings have brought these investigators to the conclusion that "illness is a state of the total organism."[33] Illness may manifest itself in several ways, usually in clusters of different symptoms; the occurrence of symptoms is related to the interpersonal relations of the individual both in his childhood and in his immediate situation.

Hinkle and his co-workers studied several groups in which extensive medical data were available over a long period of time. In two of their groups the subjects were employees of a company which had kept comprehensive health records. Considering the distribution of illnesses among the cases, they found that instead of illnesses being distributed among the subjects at random, illnesses tended to cluster more among some of the subjects than among others. Persons who had had an illness in any one body system were more likely to have an illness in another body system than persons who had had no illness.

[32] L. E. Hinkle, Jr., and H. G. Wolff, "Health and the social environment: experimental investigations," in A. Leighton, J. A. Clausen, and R. N. Wilson, eds., *Explorations in social psychiatry* (New York: Basic Books, 1957), pp. 106–32.

[33] *Ibid.*, p. 117.

The Hinkle data can be rendered in statistical terms, as follows. If illnesses were distributed among persons at random, with each illness an independent event, then the distribution of illnesses (i.e., the frequency of cases plotted against the number of illnesses per person) would be in the shape of a Poisson distribution. The Hinkle data deviate markedly from a Poisson distribution[34] in a direction which might lead one to speak of *illness-proneness*[35] as an individual characteristic. This would be analogous to the way research on accidents, in which there were similar deviations from a Poisson distribution, led the investigators to conclude that there was a specifiable characteristic associated with each individual which they called "accident proneness," and that persons differed from one another in the degree to which they were thus accident prone.[36]

[34] *Ibid.*, pp. 111–13. See a detailed discussion of the mathematics involved in L. E. Hinkle, Jr., Ruth H. Pinsky, I. D. J. Bross, and N. Plummer, "The distribution of sickness disability in a homogeneous group of 'healthy adult men,'" *American Journal of Hygiene* 64 (1956): 220–42.

[35] Hinkle *et al.* ("The distribution of sickness disability . . .") refer to differences in "general susceptibility" to illness from person to person. Additional details are also presented in L. E. Hinkle, Jr., and N. Plummer, "Life stress and industrial absenteeism: the concentration of illness and absenteeism in one segment of a working population," *Industrial Medicine and Surgery* 21 (1952): 363–75; L. E. Hinkle, Jr., and H. G. Wolff, "The nature of man's adaptation to his total environment and the relation of this to illness," *A.M.A. Archives of Internal Medicine* 99 (1957): 442–60; L. E. Hinkle, Jr., *et al.*, "An investigation of the relation between life experience, personality characteristics, and general susceptibility to illness," *Psychosomatic Medicine* 20 (1958): 278–95.

[36] M. Greenwood and Hilda Woods, *Incidence of industrial accidents upon individuals with special reference to multiple accidents*, Report No. 4 of the Industrial Fatigue Research Board (London: H. M. Stationery Office, 1919); E. M. Newbold, *A contribution to the study of the human factor in the causation of accidents*, Report No. 34 of the Industrial Fatigue Research Board (London: H. M. Stationery

Those subjects who displayed a larger number of somatic illnesses tended also to be the ones in whom psychoneuroses, psychoses, and other disturbances of thought, mood, and behavior were evident. The illnesses of those who were thus illness-prone tended to cluster in time and to coincide with periods when the individuals were having difficulty in adapting to their total life situations. Illnesses tended to occur particularly "when an individual perceives his life situation as peculiarly threatening to him."[37] The illness-prone individuals tended also to be those who "had been reared in families in which there was dissension and conflict between the parents, with hostile and rejecting attitudes on the part of one or both toward the children, divorces, emotional deprivation, and unusual restrictions or demands placed upon the offspring. Relatively few of the healthiest members of these groups had experienced any of this to a significant degree."[38] And, "it was found that during their adult lives a large proportion of the 'sickest' members . . . had experienced divorces, separations, conflict with parents, siblings, husbands and wives, uncongenial living and working arrangements, and the like and that relatively few of the healthiest members of these groups had had comparable experiences."[39]

In addition to the challenge to the doctrine of specific etiology that arises from such data as Hinkle and his as-

---

Office, 1926); E. Farmer and E. G. Chambers, *A psychological study of individual differences in accident rates*, Report No. 38 of the Industrial Fatigue Research Board (London: H. M. Stationery Office, 1926), and *A study of personal qualities in accident proneness and proficiency*, Report No. 55 of the Industrial Health Research Board (London: H. M. Stationery Office, 1929).

[37] Hinkle and Wolff, "The nature of man's adaptation to his total environment . . . ," p. 131.

[38] *Ibid.*, p. 122.   [39] *Ibid.*, p. 124.

sociates have presented, the doctrine is also challenged by the simple fact of the inexorability of death. Medical and statistical records characteristically indicate a specific "cause of death" even for the very aged. But in spite of all advances in living conditions and in methods of medical treatment, and in spite of the fact that *average* longevity has increased remarkably, the *maximum* life span has not changed at all. Old people become increasingly illness-prone and, in spite of everything, eventually die at term, as it were. Some actuarial research suggests that if all cardiovascular diseases and kidney diseases could be eliminated, only about seven or eight years would be added to the life span; and if cancer were to be eliminated, only about one to two years.[40]

Hereditary Mechanisms and Individual Survival

The doctrine of specific etiology is closely associated with another fallacious view, that *individual-survival-negative factors are all external in their locus,* that all biological mechanisms (with some few anomalous exceptions such as hemophilia) inherited by the organism essentially work *for* the individual survival of the organism and *against* insults and injuries from the outside. Within this view instances of disease and death are characteristically interpreted to indicate that the internal biological mechanisms were simply not adequate to the task of counteracting the specific etiological factor for the specific disease.

The Darwin-influenced atmosphere of our general and scientific culture lends support to the credibility of this

[40] L. I. Dublin, A. J. Lotka, and M. Spiegelman, *Length of life: a study of the life table* (New York: Ronald Press, 1949).

fallacy. Darwin explained how individual-survival-positive traits evolved. The line of thought then goes on to suggest that the very existence of a mechanism in a currently existing species is warrant that it is individual-survival-positive. The logic may be faulty, but culture, even scientific culture, is not always meticulous about logical rigor. Even before Darwin published *The origin of species* in 1859, those who had been concerned with biological mechanisms and evolution had tended to focus their attention single-mindedly on the individual-survival-positive mechanisms as if only they were "real." Individual-survival-negative mechanisms were regarded as anomalies. With the development of the Darwinian theory of natural selection, survival-negative mechanisms came to be viewed as only temporary, doomed to disappear. It is interesting that, in spite of the strongly mechanistic trend which has prevailed in biology, a trend which would consider all phenomena as equal for scientific purposes regardless of whether they seemed to be "adaptive" or "maladaptive" from the point of view of the individual, there has nonetheless been little attention paid to those features of organisms which are not individual-survival-positive. "Tooth and claw" has been given greater attention than, say, characteristics of animals which make them prey for other animals. It was precisely the positive adaptation to environment that was the starting point and major concern for Chambers in his very widely circulated and widely discussed *Vestiges of the natural history of creation* (1844), which ushered in the modern period of thought in connection with evolution.[41] The creation of individu-

---

[41] [R. Chambers,] *Vestiges of the natural history of creation*, 4th ed. (New York: Wiley and Putnam, 1846). This book was published anonymously in 1844. An interesting account of its history is presented in M. Millhauser, *Just before Darwin: Robert Chambers and*

al-survival-positive mechanisms continued to be the question to which Darwinian theory was the answer. It was the concentration on individual-survival-positive mechanisms that so strongly influenced American functionalism, as explicitly pointed out by Angell in his paper which essentially founded the school of functionalism[42] and which so strongly informed the very influential works of Cannon,[43] in which the homeostatic mechanisms were virtually single-mindedly conceived of as being on the side of individual survival.

The New Thought of Post-Darwinism, Selye, and Freud

There are three significant independent contemporary lines of thought which may be of assistance in our attempt to probe the question of the nature of disease. The first is evolutionary theory as it has developed in the past few decades. This is significant because it allows the possibility of there being individual-survival-negative factors which may be more than just anomalies to be washed out eventually by natural selection. Second, there is the line of thought developed by Selye which takes "diseases of adaptation" as its central con-

---

the Vestiges (Middletown, Conn.: Wesleyan University Press, 1959). I have dealt briefly with the relationship of Chambers to Darwin, and the relationship of these to American psychological functionalism in D. Bakan, "The influence of phrenology on American psychology," *Journal of the History of Behavioral Sciences* 2 (1966): 200–220.

[42] J. R. Angell, "The province of functional psychology," *Psychological Review* 14 (1907): 61–91; reprinted in W. Dennis, ed., *Readings in the history of psychology* (New York: Appleton-Century-Crofts, 1948), pp. 439–56.

[43] W. B. Cannon, *Bodily changes in pain, hunger, fear and rage* (New York: D. Appleton & Co., 1927), and *The wisdom of the body* (New York: W. W. Norton, 1939).

ception. The third is Freud's notion of the "death instinct" and the related considerations that he advanced. The latter two focus on individual-survival-negative mechanisms, and tend to take them as quite "natural."

In 1932 Haldane presented a new view in evolutionary theory challenging what he called the "fallacy . . . latent in most Darwinian arguments . . . that natural selection will always make an organism fitter in its struggle with the environment."[44] Simpson has summarized the point in modern evolutionary thought by saying that natural selection favors "reproductive success of a population, and nothing else." There may be instances in which reproductive success is contingent upon individual adaptation, but there is also the "possibility . . . that selection . . . could favor population reproduction at the expense of individual adaptation."[45] Although species survival may be somewhat contingent upon individual survival, natural selection may work for the survival of the species directly, and not through the intermediary of individual survival. In some species, for example, conspicuous ornamentation might be favored in sexual competition and thus increase the ornamented individual's procreative possibilities while, at the same time, that same conspicuous ornamentation might make the individual organism more visible to a predator. Furthermore, as one recent reviewer of the question has put it, "Reproduction always requires some sacrifice of resources and some jeopardy of physiological well-being, and such sacrifices may be favorably

[44] J. B. S. Haldane, *The causes of evolution* (London: Longmans, 1932), p. 119.

[45] In Anne Roe and G. G. Simpson, eds., *Behavior and evolution* (New Haven: Yale University Press, 1958), p. 20.

selected, even though they may reduce fitness in the vernacular sense of the term."[46] We cannot overlook the jeopardy to the health and very life of the mother which is associated with human childbirth. Clearly natural selection may favor the species over the individual and not, as the Darwinian mode of thought characteristically presumed, favor the species through favoring the individual.

One of the most significant developments in the modern theory of evolution is the viewpoint which has been set forth by Wynne-Edwards in his *Animal dispersion in relation to social behaviour*.[47] In his well-documented and well-argued case, he indicates that individual selection and group selection may work at cross purposes, and that the locus for the operation of the principle of natural selection is the group level. Social and group traits are largely what make for the survival of the species, but the possession of these traits may not favor the survival of the individual organism.

> What is actually passed from parent to offspring is the mechanism for responding correctly in the interest of the group in a wide range of circumstances. What is at stake is whether the group itself can survive or will become extinct. If its social adaptations prove inadequate, the stock will decline or disappear and its ground colonized by neighboring stocks with more successful systems:

[46] G. C. Williams, *Adaptation and natural selection: a critique of some current evolutionary thought* (Princeton, N. J.: Princeton University Press, 1966), p. 26. This book is an excellent summary of the current state of evolutionary thought, dealing especially with the role of natural selection.

[47] V. C. Wynne-Edwards, *Animal dispersion in relation to social behaviour* (New York: Hafner Publishing Co., 1962).

it must be by this process that group-characters slowly evolve.[48]

It is an interesting state of affairs in the history of ideas that the phenomena which provoked the theory, the individual-survival mechanisms, should somehow come under question but that the theory itself, the theory of natural selection, should be in some way hardier than the observations it was developed to explain. The characteristic assumption of Darwinian thought—that natural selection works to favor individual adaptation and thus quite automatically to favor reproductive success—is no longer tenable in this simple form. In order to understand disease we need to free our thought from the doctrine of specific etiology and from the related Pollyannaish view, associated with Darwinism, that somehow every extant mechanism in the organism works for his individual survival. Indeed a possibility which we need to be quite prepared for is that the very trait of death as a genetic characteristic of each living organism is functionally essential to the survival of the species. A "death instinct" in individuals, if it really exists, may well be in the service of the survival of the species.

Both Selye and Freud cognize constitutional factors in the organism which are not individual-survival-positive and which are, indeed, individual-survival-negative. Selye implicates "adaptation" and Freud posits an instinct to die. Paradoxical as it may appear, I suggest that *"defense" is a key notion for unlocking at least some of the mystery of the disease processes.*

In an early paper, published in 1896, Freud suggested that the efforts of the ego to "defend" itself could be

[48] *Ibid.*, p. 144.

22

regarded as the nucleus of many neuroses.[49] It would hardly be too incorrect to say that all the subsequent developments in the theory of psychoanalysis have constituted an elaboration of this one idea, certainly one of the fundamental notions of the psychoanalytic approach to personality. By virtue of the way of thinking that it suggests, neuroses may be considered quite analogous to other diseases, as the latter are conceived of by Selye. In Selye's conception, the defensive operations make up the nucleus of disease, as contrasted with the model that conceives of disease as the direct injury from external assault, whether this assault be physical or psychological. The question is raised: If the relevant mechanisms that make for disease are indeed "defense mechanisms," why is the person not defended? Why is he injured instead by the "defense mechanisms?"

Selye has examined numerous diseases of organs and systems of organs of the body and has come to the conclusion that many of them are best viewed as "diseases of adaptation,"[50] an expression which, on the face of it, appears to be composed of a pair of contradictory terms. The mechanisms that he has identified are clearly "adaptive" in much the same way as the mechanisms that Freud identified are "defensive." Yet the organism is not better adapted but, quite the contrary, is injured —in the same way as in the psychological context the individual is not better "defended" by his neurotic defense mechanisms.

[49] S. Freud, "Further remarks on the defence-psychoses," trans. J. Rickman, in *Collected papers* (London: Hogarth Press, 1950), 1: pp. 155–82.

[50] H. Selye's major treatise on this is *The physiology and pathology of exposure to stress: a treatise based on the concepts of the general-adaptation-syndrome and the diseases of adaptation* (Montreal, Canada: Acta, 1950).

The following quotation from Selye indicates the point of view to which he has been brought by his observations:

> Some diseases have specific causes, the direct actions of certain particular disease-producing agents, such as microbes, poisons, or physical injuries. Many more diseases are not caused by any one thing in particular; they result from the body's own response to some unusual situation.
>
> It is not always immediately obvious that, in the final analysis, our diseases are so often due to our own responses. . . .
>
> . . . We have seen, for instance, that if a dirty splinter of wood gets under your skin, the tissues around it swell up and become inflamed. You develop a boil or an abscess. This is a useful, healthy response, because the tissues forming the wall of this boil represent a barricade which prevents any further spread throughout the body of microbes or poisons that may have been introduced with the splinter. But sometimes the body's reactions are excessive and quite out of proportion to the fundamentally innocuous irritation to which it was exposed. Here, *an excessive response,* say, in the shape of inflammation, *may actually be the main cause of what we experience as disease.* . . . Could, for instance, the excessive production of a proinflammatory hormone, in response to some mild local irritation, result in the production of a disproportionately intensive inflammation, *which hurts more than it helps?* Could such an adaptive endocrine response become so intense that the resulting hormone-excess would damage organs in distant parts of the body, far from the original site of injury, in

parts which could not have been affected by any direct action of the external disease-producing agent?"[51]

It is quite evident that Selye has come to the conclusion that the doctrine of specific etiology is wanting and that there are mechanisms in the organism which are individual-survival-negative. The diseases that Selye considers stem from the defensive reactions to the external agent rather than from the external agent itself.

Thus Selye's observations and conclusions come remarkably close to those associated with the idea of the "death instinct," "the hypothesis that all living substance is bound to die from internal causes" which Freud explicated in *Beyond the pleasure principle*.[52] Selye has succeeded in showing in great detail how mechanisms in the organism bring about its own disease and death.

The convergence of Selye and Freud goes further than their both having recognized the existence of self-injurious mechanisms. They both also regard the nature of these mechanisms as a tendency toward a stable condition. The mechanisms that Selye points to are the same as those that Cannon called "homeostatic," which have the maintenance of a stable physiological condition as their aim. Selye's contribution has been to note that these very same mechanisms are also associated with disease and death. Freud did not have Cannon's researches available to him when he wrote of the death instinct. It is interesting, however, that he cited an early harbinger of the notion of homeostasis, "Fechner's

[51] H. Selye, *The stress of life* (New York: McGraw-Hill, 1956), pp. 128–29. Italics mine.

[52] S. Freud, *Beyond the pleasure principle*, trans. J. Strachey (New York: Liveright, 1950), p. 59.

principle of the 'tendency towards stability,' "[53] as the underlying basis for the death instinct.

Freud allowed the death instinct to be served by the self-preservative instincts. This has caused some of his readers no end of perplexity. If, however, we identify the mechanisms that he was outlining as being of the same dynamic order as the homeostatic adjustments which Selye has both identified and implicated in connection with disease and death, then this paradoxical feature of the death instinct begins to be resolved. As Cannon indicated, the homeostatic mechanisms · are clearly self-preservative. And yet, in another sense, as Selye has shown, the evidence indicates that they, in their own way, lead to disease and death. Freud wrote that "the instincts of self-preservation, of self-assertion and of mastery . . . are component instincts whose function it is to assure that the organism shall follow its own path to death, and to ward off any possible ways of returning to inorganic existence other than those which are immanent in the organism itself."[54] We think of Selye's example just cited. A barricade is produced which prevents the spread of microbes or poisons that have been introduced from the outside. But it is this very response itself, self-induced, as it were, by the organism, that is the real and dangerous disease—"immanent in the organism itself," as Freud put it.

To be sure, Freud asserted that death is a goal. In spaced type in the original German edition he said that "the goal of all life is death."[55] But ascribing goal-direction to the way in which the organism's mechanisms of defense lead to death is in no essential way different from ascribing goal-direction to the way in which the mechanisms of defense protect the organism from harm,

[53] *Ibid.*, p. 4.   [54] *Ibid.*, p. 51.   [55] *Ibid.*, p. 50.

as was, for example, done by Cannon and so magnificently captured in the title of his book *The wisdom of the body*. If—and I would like to emphasize the conditional clause here—one is justified in ascribing goal-direction when the mechanisms are individual-survival-positive, then one is *equally* justified in positing death as a goal when it can be demonstrated that the mechanisms lead to death. There may be no justification in ascribing goal-direction in either instance. But a license for the one is a license for the other. Thus, although the idea of death as a goal has been met with a certain amount of criticism by some, it should be recognized that it is no more a violation of the canons of right thinking than is "the wisdom of the body."

The agreement between Freud and Selye extends even further. Both cognized *threat of danger* as evocative of the self-injurious mechanisms. The two examples Freud used to introduce the notion of the death instinct are particularly noteworthy in that they suggest things about the nature of the death instinct which Freud did not go into very far. One example was that of a dream of a person suffering from a traumatic neurosis, in which the patient repeatedly dreams that he is back in the situation of the accident. The function of such a dream is, according to Freud, to "master the stimulus retrospectively, by developing the anxiety whose omission was the cause of the traumatic neurosis."[56] The repetition is a kind of retrospective defense against the injury. His other example is a child's game, "gone," in which the child makes things disappear and then recovers them. According to Freud this is the child's way of symbolically fortifying himself against a time when his mother might leave him, as though the act had "a defiant meaning: 'All right, then, go away! I don't need

[56] *Ibid.*, p. 39.

you. I'm sending you away myself.' "[57] It may be noted that in both instances the aim of the psychological activity is, *in a certain sense*, protection from injury but in neither instance is there specific real protection against injury. In the one example the trauma is not averted by dreaming of the accident; in the other example the mother is not prevented from leaving the child. Nonetheless, both the dream and the child's game are, in this certain limited sense of the term, *defensive*. Freud might have said, had he discussed the meaning of his examples more fully, that the death instinct, which they are supposed to exemplify, is manifested precisely in "defenses" which do not defend, which injure, and which nonetheless *appear* to defend from injury.

It is also of more than parenthetical interest that the examples Freud saw fit to use to illustrate the death instinct should have involved the two major kinds of suffering, suffering through physical injury and suffering through loss of loved ones, the two afflictions of Job.

The processes associated with self-injury are conceived of in the writings of Freud and Selye as having extremely wide compass, as including inflictions which ordinarily would not be thought of as due to the responses of the organism itself. In the passage from Selye quoted above, he clearly says that "in the final analysis, our diseases are so often due to our own responses," more often, it would seem, than from external injury—and he at times indicates that external injury can often also be traced to actions of the individual himself. Freud similarly indicated that the "ultimate cause of the death of all higher organisms" is that they die from "products of" their "own metabolism."[58]

The death instinct, according to Freud, is evident in

[57] *Ibid.*, p. 15. [58] *Ibid.*, p. 65.

the *compulsion to repeat*, which he variously describes as "primitive," "elementary," and "instinctual," the "manifestations" of which "give the appearance of some extraneous force at work."[59] The fact that he attributes the compulsion to repeat to the death instinct may help us to explicate the nature of the mechanism involved in disease somewhat better. It should be observed that every neurosis is characterized by the compulsion to repeat. Neurosis may be defined as a condition in which some regular response occurs in the individual in spite of his conscious wish that he not make that response. In obsessions, phobias, and compulsions, the classical forms of neurosis, the individual has thoughts or fears, or engages in acts in opposition to his conscious intentions, and even to his disadvantage. The responses indeed appear to occur as though there were "some extraneous force at work." It is precisely this *automatic* occurrence, occurrence independent of the conscious ego, that marks the response as neurotic. The way in which events take place *automatically* in the organism is what Freud identified as reflecting the work of the death instinct. Now, when we read Selye describing how physiological reactions are triggered quite automatically, resulting in the injury of the organism, we are led to the opinion that automatic defense processes constitute the major factor in disease and death. Both Freud's death instinct and Selye's diseases of adaptation may be identified with those automatic mechanisms in the organism, the primitive, elementary, and instinctual mechanisms, which are phenomenologically extraneous to the conscious ego.

There is a paradox in Freud's thought which these considerations may help us resolve, as well as help us to come closer to understanding some of the mystery of

[59] *Ibid.*, p. 45.

disease. Freud suggested an identification of the death
instinct with the ego instincts,[60] albeit with qualifica
tion. Yet he had an ideal which he expressed as, "Where
id was there shall ego be."[61] It should be noted that the
mechanisms associated with self-injury are, on the one
hand, both phenomenologically alien to the ego and (in
a certain sense) self-preservative. Yet, on the other
hand, it is also evident that they are self-injurious. How
could the injuriousness associated with the mechanisms
be mitigated? Clearly, the way to overcome the injuriousness of a mechanism is to change that which is ego-
alien to something which is not ego-alien, to recognize
that that which may have the sense of being "other" (as
the word "id" so strongly suggests) is really the person
himself, to overcome the automaticity of the functioning
of such mechanisms that have only the *appearance of defense* so that indeed the person may be really defended
instead of injured by them.

Selye is hardly a trained psychologist or psychiatrist.
Nonetheless his findings lead him to at least one aspect
of the psychoanalytic position, that there is a relationship between self-knowledge and therapy. His advice is
"know thyself,"[62] essentially the advice of all psychoanalysis. He aptly characterizes emotional defense responses associated with disease as manifestations of a
person's being in a situation where he is protecti ng
himself from being "done in."[63] In order to overcome
the disease processes he suggests bringing to bear the
"mechanisms of surrender," that one may possibly turn
the tide of the disease process by encouraging the body

[60] *Ibid.*, p. 58.

[61] S. Freud, *New introductory lectures to psychoanalysis*, trans.
W. J. H. Sprott (New York: W. W. Norton, 1933), p. 112.

[62] *The stress of life*, pp. 260 ff.

[63] *Ibid.*, p. 262.

"not to defend itself"—interesting advice based on the recognition that the defense mechanisms are more injurious than assault from the outside. Whether such simple exhortation can be therapeutic is an empirical question. But Selye is quite convinced that *"knowing what hurts you has an inherent curative value"*[64]—to which I would add—if it overcomes the automaticity of response.

The Paradox of Telic Decentralization

At this point it will profit our discussion to introduce for serious consideration the notion of telos. I have already touched upon it in indicating the goal-direction feature associated with both the notion of homeostasis and the notion of the death instinct, although, as will be evident, literal purpose as known in consciousness need not be presumed in the notion of telos. Among the major and recurrent issues in the field of biology that of mechanistic versus telic explanation of biological phenomena characteristically comes to the fore when what ultimately concerns man is under discussion. One of the significant features of the Darwinian theory of evolution is that it provided a way of explaining evolution without any notion of telos, of explaining, as someone once said, how it might be possible to build a house just by throwing bricks. Unfortunately, the Darwinian theory of evolution is intrinsically unconfirmable because it is a historical hypothesis. Historical hypotheses are all intrinsically unconfirmable. This is not to say that evidences cannot be brought forth which increase or decrease the tenability of any historical hypothesis. Nor should this observation detract from the greatness of

[64] *Ibid.*, p. 260.

the Darwinian theory. But insofar as a hypothesis concerns history it cannot be directly confirmed. The intrinsic impossibility is the logical consequence of the very meanings of the words "history" and "confirm."

I would like to draw further on the thought of Selye in connection with what he has to say about telos. In an effort to reconcile the seeming "purposefulness" of the mechanisms which he has observed with the evident fact that they also make for disease and death, he has suggested the notion of multiple *teleologic centers*, especially that that which is purposeful with respect to one center may not be so for the total organism:

> All my factual observations were made possible by experiments planned on the assumption that stress-responses are purposeful, homeostatic reactions. We must realize that in both the examples just mentioned (inflammation in response to microbes and cancer) there are actually two *teleologic centers;* their interests are opposed but, within each of them, purposeful activity "for its own good" is clearly recognizable. On the one hand is the interest of the patient, on the other that of the microbe or of the cancer. Indeed, the very essence of cancerous growth is the setting up of a center whose own interests are largely opposed to those of its host.[65]

Thus, following Selye, instead of attempting to resolve the question of mechanism versus teleology in any ultimate sense, let us instead consider the possibility that in the healthy organism there is a higher telos tending to dominate all lower telê, and that *disease is to be conceived of as decentralization of this higher telos of the organism, and its loss of dominance over the lower telê.*

[65] *Ibid.*, p. 245.

32

Consider the following example. Ordinarily there is very limited proliferation of the cells of the skin. When there is damage to the skin, however, the cells next to the damaged area undergo proliferation. Capillaries grow into the region where the regeneration is taking place. When regeneration is complete, proliferation ceases. Detailed analysis of the nature of the underlying biochemical processes may be made. Yet, no matter how detailed or extensive such an analysis may be, it cannot quite get at the fact that the end product of whatever biochemical processes may be involved is still regenerated skin. The mechanisms that lead to various types of form-determination are multiple; and the recognition of the multiple ways by which living organisms arrive at similar or identical forms has led a vitalistic thinker such as Driesch to speak of *equifinality* as a way of comprehending the data. The development of embryos and the regeneration of injured tissue usually take place in specific step-by-step processes. If there is interference with the normal processes, however, organisms often, although not always, display remarkable ingenuity and deviousness to come to the same or a functionally similar end by different processes. For any given level of form-determination we may speak of that which determines the form, whatever its ultimate nature may be, as the telos.

Biological entities may be considered as being composed of various levels of organization, constituting a *hierarchical order*.[66] Form exists on every level, even though the form at any particular level consists of components of a lower level of the hierarchical order. The form at any one level is not the necessary logical consequence of form at a lower level. At each level there ap-

[66] See J. H. Woodger, *Biological principles* (London: Routledge and Kegan Paul, 1948), pp. 311–17.

pears to be *something*, whatever it may be, which organizes the components of the next lower level. *Telos may be simply defined as "determinant of form."* Such notions as entelechy, Bergson's *élan vital*, and McDougall's *hormé* suggest themselves as similar to this notion of telos. Although this "something" to which I here allude is certainly that which these terms denote, each of them is also part of a connotative, and a further denotative, complex with which I do not necessarily want to involve my present thesis.

The meaning of telic decentralization as a way of conceptualizing disease may be made clearer by considering what we ordinarily refer to as *communication*, since telic decentralization involves a reduction in communication. In a general sense everyone knows what conscious communication is. It is manifest in two people talking to each other in such a way that the second person becomes conscious of that which the first person was conscious of initially. The kinds of observation arising from psychoanalysis illustrate another kind of communication, the kind of internal communication that takes place when something of which the individual had been unconscious becomes conscious in him without its having been communicated to him by another person. Within the human organism there are varieties of forms of communication evident when what happens in one part of the body affects what happens in other parts. There are numerous mechanisms in such internal communication, the neural and hormonal being particularly conspicuous. But biological communication is more general than any of the particular communication mechanisms that have been identified. The mechanisms are remarkably diverse. The fact that communication takes place, by whatever mechanism, pervades all biological phenomena. Conscious communication between

34

persons may be regarded as a particular instance of the more general communication that occurs. But consciousness, as such, is not the essential ingredient of communication.

Let us consider an example used by Sinnott to explicate the nature of biological development of form, the cellular slime mold. This organism starts with a single cell which continues to divide until there are numerous such cells. They mill around freely for some time. After a period the movement of the cells in the mass stops. Some cells at the bottom anchor themselves and become a disk. Other cells in the center develop thick walls, adhere to each other and to the disk, and form a stalk. The remaining cells, still in free motion, go up the stalk and form a body at the top. Each of the cells at the top forms a spore, dries up, and is blown away, capable of beginning all over again to multiply by cell division, form a disk, stalk, etc. Sinnott comments on this as follows:

> The morphogenetic mechanism that operates here is very hard to understand. Individual cells are certainly alike. None seems to have any predetermined position in the whole. Each can become a disk cell, a stalk cell, or a spore, depending on its position. One may argue that the individual cells are the final factors and that what takes place is the result of subtle and specific differences in contact and chemical attraction between them resulting in a specific pattern, but it is very difficult to see how this is brought about. In some way the cells become different as they take up different positions in the whole. As Vöchting and Driesch pointed out many years ago, the fate of a cell is a function of its position. But, it may be asked, its

35

position in *what?* Here one is confronted by the ancient question as to whether the cell of the organized cellular system is the ultimate biological unity; whether an organic form is the result of chemical and physical interactions between independent units, the cells; or whether, when these cells are in contact with one another, there is set up some such factor as a differential diffusion pattern in the cytoplasm, a bio-electrical field, or some other formative influence that unites the cells into a formed whole.[67]

In some way the fact that one cell has become part of the disk is communicated to other cells which become stalk, and this information is in turn communicated to still other cells which become spores. Whatever the mechanism may be, it can be presumed that there is some mechanism of intercellular communication working to produce the total form, a mechanism to which we need not ascribe consciousness but which is telic by our notion.

Consider some data from another source. It has been demonstrated that when normal tissues are grown on a glass surface, the cells stop growing when they touch each other. But cancer cells similarly grown on a glass surface continue to grow, unimpeded by cellular contact. Loewenstein and his associates at Columbia University have attempted to probe this phenomenon by the technique of passing a current of ions into a cell and assessing the current leak which prevails in the adjacent cell. They believe that the cessation of growth on contact in normal cells means "Some kind of signal must be

[67] E. W. Sinnott, *The problem of organic form* (New Haven: Yale University Press, 1963), pp. 21–22. For a general treatment of the development of slime molds, see J. T. Bonner, *The cellular slime molds* (Princeton, N.J.: Princeton University Press, 1959).

transmitted from cell to cell on contact."[68] They have found that such electrical measurements in adjacent cells are negligible among cancer cells as contrasted with substantially higher measurements in adjacent cells for corresponding normal tissues. "The differences in functional communication are so marked that they offer a means for identifying cancer with ease at the cellular level."[69] If ionic transfer may be looked upon as the means of communication among cells, then, as Loewenstein and his associates maintain, "Cancer cells are . . . unable to engage in the kind of communication possible in their normal counterparts."[70]

The telos of a particular level of the organizational hierarchy is clearly contingent on communication, whatever the detailed mechanisms of communication may be, among the components at a lower level. It turns out that the cells of cancer, which are radically and manifestly removed from the telos of any higher level of the hierarchical order, are precisely those cells which are distinguishable from their cellular counterparts by a gross inability to communicate with other cells, as indicated both by their growth behavior and by the lack of ionic transfer.

[68] W. R. Loewenstein and Y. Kanno, "Intercellular communication and the control of tissue growth: lack of communication between cancer cells," *Nature* 209 (1966): 1248–49.

[69] *Ibid.*, p. 1249.

[70] *Ibid.* The general theory of the role of ions in intercellular communication and relevant experimentation are reported in the following papers: W. R. Loewenstein, S. J. Socolar, S. Higashino, Y. Kanno, and N. Davidson, "Intercellular communication: renal, urinary bladder, sensory and salivary gland cells," *Science* 149 (1965): 295–98; W. R. Loewenstein and Y. Kanno, "Studies on an epithelial (gland) cell junction. I. Modifications of surface membrane permeability," *Journal of Cell Biology* 22 (1964): 565–86; J. Wiener, D. Spiro, and W. R. Loewenstein, "Studies on an epithelial (gland) cell junction. II. Surface structure," *Journal of Cell Biology* 22 (1964): 587–98.

But now let us think back to the data and conclusions of Hinkle and his associates which have already been cited. Their findings indicate that the condition of being ill is a general characteristic of the total organism and that the particular form that the illness takes is secondary. A person with any one illness is more likely to get another disease, even in a remote body system, than a person who has had no illness. Furthermore, the evidences brought forth by these investigators, as well as by other studies cited earlier, indicate that persons who suffer somatic illnesses are persons who also tend to manifest psychological disorders. Some people are more illness-prone than others. Illness-proneness varies with the time in one's life. Illness-proneness is associated with psychological condition. Illness-proneness is associated with the experience of threat. Now, if repression is a major factor in psychological disorders as Freud asserted, and if, say, repression is a manifestation in the psyche of organismic telic decentralization, it may then be said that *a degree of telic decentralization is the essential underlying characteristic of the diseased organism.*

Telic and Psychological Processes

As I have already suggested, it is important that we distinguish between telos and conscious purpose. Processes may be said to be telic insofar as they are determined by whatever it is that determines form at a particular level of organization. The lower the level of functioning in the hierarchical order, the less do the processes suggest that anything like conspicuous purpose is operative. In the case of the human being there emerges something which is manifestly, consciously, phenomenologically, and introspectively evident, namely, purpose as deliberate. The anti-teleological biologists have a deep —and valid—aversion to the ascription of anything like conscious or deliberate purpose to processes at lower levels; they prefer "built up" rather than "built down" explanations of biological events. But let us conscientiously reserve the term "telos" exclusively for the influence determining form, and the term "purpose" for the conscious determination of form by the human being. If we accept this distinction, it is evident that purpose is conscious telos. The anti-teleological biologists are correct in refusing to attribute purpose to lower levels of biological form. One cannot, however, reasonably deny the reality and significance of telos at lower levels.

Let us return to a consideration of psychoanalysis for a possible illumination of the nature of telos. Freud asserted that in the formation of a dream there is an underlying wish; yet the wish is not recognized by the individual. It is wrong to call such a wish a purpose precisely because it is unconscious. The significance of Freud's observation lies in its indication of the existence of telê operative in the human psyche which are not consciously recognized purposes. The neurosis exists because there are such telê in the psyche and because, furthermore, they are functionally separated from, and not under the control of, conscious purposes. It is the separation of these telê from purpose that brings about the neurotic condition, the disease, of the individual. Psychoanalytic therapy can be conceived of as an attempt to bring these telê under the dominion of the conscious purposes of the psyche and thus to overcome the telic decentralization involved in the existence of such separated lower telê.

The notion of telos places us in a better position to appreciate Freud's strange identification between the instincts of self-preservation and the death instinct. We may clarify the paradox that the very mechanisms associated with growth and development and survival of the individual are at one and the same time the mechanisms which lead to death: *In multicellular organisms the formation of lower, subsidiary telê constitutes an essential feature of growth and development.* From the moment of the first division of the fertilized cell there is decentralization of the central telos of the organism into the telê of organs and systems; unless each organ or system has a telos which is, to some degree, decentralized, the organ or system cannot function effectively as part of the total organism. *The basic paradox is that organismic growth and development can take place only if there is a certain degree of telic decentralization, while at the same time disease and death also result from such telic decentralization.* As we have learned from Selye's work, disease often occurs when the mechanism of "adaptation," which would indeed be adaptive if it were still functioning in accordance with the higher telos of the organism, begins to function "for its own good," as Selye puts it.

Insofar as there is telic decentralization, to that extent do the processes become automatic and "mechanistic." The central telos of the organism is manifested most clearly in the conscious purposes of a differentiated organism. As I have suggested, the natural tendency in the psyche toward telic decentralization may be identified with what the psychoanalysts refer to as repression. In seeking an understanding of disease and death we are thus brought to a further consideration of the nature of the psyche.

To do this, there is some value in considering the theoretical notion of isomorphism, which has been advanced most explicitly by the Gestalt school of psychology.[71] It is maintained that the essential form of a stimulus object in perception is repeated on both the psychological and the physiological levels. The stress of the Gestalt school has been largely on the isomorphism of stimulus and physiology. Clear-cut empirical data to substantiate this particular form of isomorphism have been hard to come by. The concept has received little widespread attention among psychologists in recent years.

If we turn our attention to another pair of the isomorphic trio, however, the psychological and the physiological levels (excluding the stimulus object), there appears to be more to commend isomorphism to our attention. Gotthard Booth, for example, has found that the Rorschach responses of cancer patients tend to be highly differentiated into isolated organisms or objects. There is also an unusual lack of apprehension of symmetry in the ink blots. These responses are remarkably suggestive of the formal physical characteristics of cancer itself.[72] Fisher and Cleveland have been able to demonstrate clear-cut isomorphisms between Rorschach responses and different categories of disease, including rheumatoid arthritis, neurodermatitis, stomach disorders, spastic colitis, and cancer. In one of their studies, for example, distinct differences in Rorschach patterns were demonstrated between patients with exterior cancers (e.g., breast) and patients with interior cancers (e.g., cervix). The former had substantially higher "barrier" scores on the Rorschach, whereas the latter had lower "barrier" scores and higher "penetration" scores.[73]

[71] See K. Koffka, *Principles of Gestalt psychology* (New York: Harcourt, Brace, 1935), pp. 56 ff.

[72] G. Booth, "Irrational complications of the cancer problem," *American Journal of Psychoanalysis* 25 (1965): 41–60.

[73] S. Fisher and S. E. Cleveland, *Body image and personality* (Princeton, N.J.: D. Van Nostrand, 1958), p. 304.

It is part of normal development that *both* the ego and the body should develop, and that the isomorphism be imperfect. In the very development of the organism there arises both the discernment of the body from the rest of the world and the discernment of the ego from the body, although there are special relationships among the three. Freud wrote in *The ego and the id*, "The ego is first and foremost a body-ego; it is not merely a surface entity, but it is itself the projection of a surface." To this assertion the translator has added the following comment, "I.e., the ego is ultimately derived from bodily sensations, chiefly from those springing from the surface of the body. It may thus be regarded as a mental projection of the surface of the body, besides, as we have seen above, representing the superficies of the mental apparatus."[74]

In any number of instances psychoanalysts have allowed themselves to interpret words describing actions of the body in terms of their metaphorical significance, as though psychological and physical forms of functioning are one. This practice is evident, for example, in Erikson's identification of body *zone* with psychological *mode*. Thus, for example, "The anal-urethral sphincters, then, are the anatomic models for the *retentive* and *eliminative* modes, which, in turn, can characterize a great variety of behaviors."[75]

Such considerations suggest that a close examination of the nature of the psyche may perhaps give us some hint concerning the fate of the telos in the organism, and may even give us some understanding of the nature of the physiological processes involved. We must do this

[74] S. Freud, *The ego and the id*, trans. Joan Riviere (London: Hogarth Press, 1950), p. 31.

[75] E. H. Erikson, *Childhood and society*, 2d ed. (New York: W. W. Norton, 1963), p. 52.

quite gingerly, since we really have no guarantee that the psychological really would invariably follow the physical.

But perhaps to note the formal features of the psyche might offer some suggestions for winning a better understanding of disease and death. This is what Freud did in his further elaboration of the death instinct in *The ego and the id;* here he indicated that he would not draw from biology any longer (as he had done earlier in *Beyond the pleasure principle*) but would stay closer to psychoanalysis.

Freud took great pains to show that within the ego there were unconscious forces. He identified repression as a function of the ego, even though the process was unconscious. If we can translate the insight that Freud manifested into the terms which we have been developing, it appears that there are forces within the psyche which are themselves unconscious and which lead to the decentralization of the telos. In some sense this is captured by the term "id," that which is yet a part of the individual psyche but which has the appearance of being "it," and "not me." Thus the very psyche itself gets separated into "it" and "me." This particular separation is especially significant for our appreciation of the meaning of pain; but we must reserve that for the next chapter.

Freud identified the superego as part of the ego, but at the same time unconscious. Especially in the case of melancholia, which Freud understood as the result of loss (and we should remind ourselves of the data cited on the relationship between various forms of separation-estrangement and disease), "the super-ego can become a kind of gathering place for the death-instincts,"[76]

[76] *The ego and the id*, p. 79.

"holding sway in the super-ego is, as it were, a pure culture of the death-instinct, and in fact it often enough succeeds in driving the ego into death."[77]

Translating this into our terms, the superego is formed and a force emerges from the superego which leads to further decentralization of the telos. But Freud also understood the superego to be associated with threat; and Selye too regards threat as a major factor in creating the "diseases of adaptation." According to Selye we have stress leading to the decentralization of the telos, with the adaptive mechanism running on its own, "for its own good," but leading to disease and death. On the psychological level we have the ego, the major telic center. Associated with it are the forces toward repression. Threat is conceptualized as embodied in the superego. The superego is part of the ego. Neurosis is largely the result of the action of the superego. Thus, as we have already indicated, both Selye and Freud bring us to the same consequent: the individual gets sick from immanent forces, forces which can be triggered by threat and which run off automatically outside the dominion of conscious control. In some sense exactly the same processes are being examined, Freud looking at them from above and Selye from below. The works of Selye and Freud have pointed up the fact that every person has a fatal disease, the decentralization of the telos, from which he must eventually die.

What is disease in one instance makes for growth and development in another. In Chapter III, I will develop in some detail a line of thought stimulated by reading the Book of Job. Anticipating that line of thought, consider death as the inevitable consequent of having been born; and the possibility that in the face of the inevitability of death, dying *deferentially* arises as a

[77] *Ibid.*, p. 77.

psychological mechanism. We have an instance of the self responding to threat by *deferring* to the threatening situation in Freud's example of the game of "gone," in which the child arrogates to himself the leaving of the mother in the face of the threat that she will actually leave him. In the example of the dream of the accident we also have an instance in which psychologically the individual is doing to himself what had been done to him, subjecting himself again and again to the circumstances surrounding his injury. It is, after all, *his* dream. Physiologically and psychologically the reaction to threat is deference on the part of the organism, the organism doing to itself what the external situation is threatening to do to it—to injure and possibly to kill it. Freud's writings explained this self-injury as deference to an internalized father-figure who punishes the ego from the inside of the ego as the father might have punished the child from the outside. Selye's writings certainly do not indicate concern with deference in the psychological sense. Yet at the same time what he has outlined as the nature of the mechanisms in the diseases of adaptation constitutes deference, at least in a certain formal sense—the arousal of self-injurious processes in response to external threat. In any circumstances, if threat is responded to by self-injury it is certainly *as though* disease and death were deferential, whether experienced as such or not.

But, then, Freud did not purport to describe conscious experience. On the contrary, the mechanisms of guilt and self-injury that he speaks of are precisely those mechanisms which are unconscious, which we have taken as telic but not purposeful and have interpreted as removed from the central telos of the organism. Selye's research reports constitute a description of the physiological substrata of deferential self-injury.

In psychoanalytic literature there is often a systematic refusal to honor the distinction between aggression directed toward oneself and that directed against another. Some of the validity in so refusing to honor the distinction between self and other becomes evident when we recognize the mechanisms of deferential self-injury prevailing both psychologically and physiologically, and the way in which these mechanisms are triggered by threat.

Telos and Eros

This brings us to a reconsideration of the notion of Eros developed by Freud in *Beyond the pleasure principle*. In that essay Freud conceived of the multicellular quality of organisms as one of their most significant characteristics. Eros tries "to combine organic substances into ever larger unities."[78] It "binds all living things together."[79] It "seeks to force together and hold together the portions of living substance."[80] What Freud was referring to by the term Eros apparently was what Sinnott meant by a "formative influence that unites the cells into a formed whole," as indicated in the passage quoted above, and what we are calling telos. If we allow such an identification, it suggests that we might go a little further with Freud on the notion of Eros as also the force associated with the making of larger human group formations and general interpersonal relations, as indeed Freud actually suggested in *Group psychology and the analysis of the ego*.[81]

[78] *Beyond the pleasure principle*, p. 57.

[79] *Ibid.*, p. 68.   [80] *Ibid.*, p. 84.

[81] S. Freud, *Group psychology and the analysis of the ego*, trans. J. Strachey (London: Hogarth Press, 1949).

Freud indicated on several occasions that transference was a prerequisite for effective psychoanalytic therapy. If a strong emotional relationship with at least one person could be established, then repression within the individual might be overcome. I believe that Freud had here a profound intuition about the relationship between the intrapsychic and the social. If the isolation of the individual from the larger *social telos* could be overcome, if contact and communication between the individual and at least one other person in the larger social body could be established, the person might be healed. In other words, if the social telos could again be brought into play so as to integrate the individual organism into the larger society, the latter equally conceived of as an organism, the telic decentralization within the organism might be overcome.

There have been numerous instances in which psychotherapy has been used effectively in the treatment of somatic conditions. Let us briefly consider a study conducted by a group of investigators at the Columbia-Presbyterian Medical Center. The investigators studied and compared two groups of patients suffering from ulcerative colitis for a period of seven years. Both groups received routine medical treatment. Each group consisted of fifty-seven patients, the groups having been matched on the basis of severity of illness, sex, age of onset of the illness, and the use of steroid therapy. One group was treated with psychotherapy or psychoanalysis, the precise form of psychological treatment being dictated by the nature of the case. The other group received no psychological therapy. Regular physical examinations, conducted independently of any psychological treatment, were made on all patients, and systematic ratings of proctoscopic observations and symptoms were recorded. It was found that "the [psychotherapeutically] treated group showed a marked and sustained improvement while the control group remained relatively status quo," leading these investigators to conclude that "there is a definite role for psychotherapy in the treatment of ulcerative colitis."[82]

The belief that interpersonal warmth might be a factor in clinical progress has affected nursing programs and nursing education. In one study a clear relationship has been shown between the kind of attention given to the patient prior to surgery and the amount of postoperative vomiting. Patients who were systematically and conscientiously helped by a nurse to attain what the investigators referred to as a "suitable psychological state for surgery," by inquiry into the causes of distress and efforts to relieve the distress, accompaniment by the nurse to the operating room and table, and so on, showed a substantially (and statistically significant) lower incidence of postoperative vomiting: 16 per cent of the experimental group compared to 54 per cent of the control group. The control group received routine preoperative care.[83]

A similar approach has been tried in an interesting experimental program of nursing at the Loeb Center of the Montefiore Hospital in New York City. Here a carefully worked out program of nursing includes around-the-clock psychological and emotional care of patients in addition to routine medical and bodily care. The nurses are trained in psychotherapy, largely based on the non-directive approach of Carl Rogers. The aim of

[82] J. F. O'Connor, G. Daniels, A. Karush, L. Moses, C. Flood, and Lenore O. Stein, "The effects of psychotherapy on the course of ulcerative colitis: a preliminary report," *American Journal of Psychiatry* 120 (1964): 741.

[83] Rhetaugh G. Dumas and R. C. Leonard, "The effect of nursing on the incidence of postoperative vomiting," *Nursing Research* 12 (1963): 12–15.

the nursing treatment is to help the patient understand himself and his problems. The nurses do not wear uniforms. Each nurse has only eight patients during waking hours, which in effect means that she can spend an hour a day on the average with each patient. Each nurse is also provided with a messenger-attendant (one per two nurses) whose job is to run various errands, thus maximizing the time that the nurse actually spends with the patients.

The actual times between admission and discharge in this program have run substantially below physicians' predictions.[84] In one group of 250 patients, only 9 were readmitted to hospitals within a year of discharge, less than 4 per cent, compared to the usual 18 per cent readmission rate for comparable groups of patients.[85]

Observations such as these suggest that such efforts as man can devise and apply to overcome telic decentralization on the social level can work against the processes associated with disease and death, although they cannot overcome the inexorability of the latter.

Some Concluding Comments

Telic decentralization is essential to growth, development, and reproduction, as is telic centralization. And yet, paradoxically, the continuation of telic decentrali-

[84] Genrose Alfano and Estelle Bernardin, "Can nursing care hasten recovery?" *American Journal of Nursing* 64 (June, 1964): 80–85. See also Lydia E. Hall and Genrose Alfano, "The patient with myocardial infarction: incapacitation or rehabilitation?" *American Journal of Nursing* 64 (November, 1964): C-20–C-25; Lydia E. Hall, "A center for nursing," *Nursing Outlook* 11 (November, 1963): 805–6; and "Summary of Project: Loeb Center for Nursing and Rehabilitation," June, 1963, mimeographed.

[85] Personal communication from Mrs. Lydia E. Hall, Director of the Loeb Center.

zation leads to the ultimate death of the individual organism. Freud indicated in *Beyond the pleasure principle* that the death instinct was primitively located in the individual cell, and that the existence of multicellular organisms emerged only as a result of the additional Eros. He accepted the Weismann notion that the organism consisted of soma and germ plasm, adding that the death instinct resided in the soma whereas Eros lived in the germ plasm. He conceptualized ejaculation in the male as associated with the death instinct but saw the coalescence of germ cells as associated with life instincts. Thus, whatever involves the separation of cells is of the death instinct, but whatever is associated with conjugation, coalescence, cohesion, coordination, or communication among cells is of Eros. Freud rather arbitrarily asserted that the death instinct was older than the life instinct. If we accept the view that life was originally formed as a one-celled organism, then it certainly could be said that the death instinct is older than the life instinct.

An identification of the death instinct with the fundamental tendency of organisms to divide into separate living entities as in fission is certainly suggested by Freud. The aim of dividing and the aim of dying indeed do not appear to be the same. Yet they are the same in the sense that after fission the parent cell no longer exists as a unitary organism. Thus we have the problem of the definition of death that Freud struggled with briefly in *Beyond the pleasure principle*. Should one accept the view of Goette that death is the direct result of reproduction?[86] Or Hartmann, that death is not the appearance of a dead body but the termination of individual development?[87] Fission is the paradigmatic form of

[86] *Beyond the pleasure principle*, p. 63.
[87] *Ibid.*

telic decentralization; and, so conceived, it is unnecessary to assume the additional burden of having to assert and defend the notion that death is a goal, as Freud unfortunately did. Death may, however, yet be an important mechanism for the survival of the species.

There are the familiar stages of birth, childhood, puberty, adolescence, adulthood, old age, and death. Telic decentralization processes take place throughout all the stages, although in the early stages they are more often identifiable as growth and in the later stages as disease and finally death itself. Death occurs because the fission-like processes continue, and continue beyond a point where they are coordinated by the telos of the total organism. As fission of a one-celled organism necessarily entails the annihilation of the organism, so may fission-like processes be associated with the annihilation of the multicellular organism. The organism is endowed at birth with the tendency toward the decentralization of the telos. If it were not for this there would be no growth and development. Although necessary for growth and development, however, the same tendency leads to disease and death.

The human organism is both strongly individualistic, separated from other organisms, and strongly social, involved in a larger human telos. Both these characteristics inhere in his particular developmental pattern. There is the very long period between his birth and his ability to reproduce. In his early childhood he is extremely dependent on others for the maintenance of life. In the long period between early childhood and adolescence, the period referred to in psychoanalytic literature as the latency period, he is generally involved in the development of strongly individualistic patterns. There is also the very long period between the time at which reproduction is no longer possible and maximum longev-

51

ity. Indeed, one may speculate that the latter is functionally related to the former. For if children need long care after birth, there is also a need for parents to give them that care, long enough after their capability of producing new organisms has ceased. And perhaps the greater longevity of the female, and her generally more delayed tendency toward telic decentralization, manifested, for example, in her greater resistance to degenerative diseases, is equally related to the fact that children need long care—but this is speculation and one would need more data to make such an argument cogent.

The many human beings in the world seem to be all part of the larger telos associated with their common ancestry. In the same way, as in the example of the slime mold cited earlier, all the thousands of cells resulting from a single cell tend to participate in a way which indicates that there is a "formative influence" among them, so may there be some single telos among all human beings. The same set of factors that make for man's differentiation into a single individual, a single person, also make for his ultimate death. At the same time there must be a larger telos of which he is a part, the cultivation of which may make it possible for him to lengthen the life that he has (within maximum limits), to live to a great age as did, presumably, Abraham and Job. Some of the evidence which has been cited seems to indicate that telic decentralization works downward, from a higher level of biological organization to the point of utmost telic decentralization of which the disease we call cancer is the extreme example. We have also seen that there are some degrees of freedom associated with man at the psychological level and the societal level whereby he can, by the increase of understanding and the increase of communication, maintain telic centralization at the higher levels of biological organization. Man may not be able to make himself, as an individual, immortal. But it is within his power to extend his life within the larger societal telos. By working to maintain the larger telos he may increase the number of his days as well.

I I

Pain
and the Functions
of the Ego

MY heart is sore pained within me:
and the terrors of death
are fallen upon me.
Fearfulness and trembling
are come upon me,
and horror hath overwhelmed me.
PSALM 55:4–5

*I*N THIS chapter I shall attempt to advance some lines of thought whereby the phenomenon of pain may be conceptualized. I have thus far dealt with human suffering through the consideration of disease. Pain and disease are, of course, intimately related. The separation of one from the other for expository purposes is necessarily in violation of the substantive matter under discussion. The only warrant would be the possibility that clarity may be served by the separation. Thus let us consider with greater directness that most dramatic and conspicuous form of suffering which we call pain.

Pain and the Meaning of Life

Pain is the common companion of birth and growth, disease and death, and is a phenomenon deeply intertwined with the very question of human existence. It is among the most salient of human experiences; and it often precipitates questioning the meaning of life itself.

To attempt to understand the nature of pain, to seek to find its meaning, is already to respond to an imperative of pain itself. No experience demands and insists upon interpretation in the same way. Pain forces the question of its meaning, and especially of its cause, insofar as cause is an important part of its meaning. In those instances in which pain is intense and intractable and in which its causes are obscure, its demand for interpretation is most naked, manifested in the sufferer asking, "Why?" Thus, our very effort to understand the nature of pain is natural, much as it is natural for man to concern himself with disease.

Pain has a significant place in a number of world views which attempt to give meaning to our experiences. In the hedonistic world views, pain, together with what is sometimes regarded as its counterpart, pleasure, has been taken as basic to human experience, as a phenomenon from which other experiences and phenomena derive. In the thought of a number of classical social theorists—Bentham, Adam Smith, and others—pain is a given and constitutes the basis for explaining the complex interactions of men and their arrangements. Furthermore, systematic infliction of pain on others is the major function of some of our important social institutions, such as police and armies, and a major function even of the family, school, and church.

Pain has played a central role in the religious thought of Western civilization. For her disobedience in the Garden of Eden, Eve is condemned to bring forth children in sorrow (Gen. 3:16); and the central image in the history of the Western world has been that of a crucifixion, undoubtedly one of the most painful forms of execution ever devised. I regard it as indicative of something important in both the mind of man and the nature of our culture that the dominant image in the history of Western civilization has been that of one obviously suffering pain. Pain must, in some sense, be a touchstone for ultimate concern. It is also noteworthy that in spite of all other differences many of our secular philosophies and our religious tradition should converge in giving pain a central place.

Although the phenomena associated with pain are remarkably complex, the major thesis of this chapter may be stated rather simply. *Pain is the psychic manifestation of telic decentralization.*

Pain, Science, and Individual Experience

The individual person, insofar as he is an individual, is already to a large degree decentralized from the larger social telos. Pain and autonomous individual existence are linked in a certain inexorable manner. Pain does not exist until there is an organism which has been individuated. Pain can, indeed, be taken as the characterizing experience of the human organism torn out of a larger telos, seen so clearly, for example, in the cry of a child at birth—the critical individuating experience, as was recognized by Rank.[1]

The very quandaries associated with the effort to study pain from a scientific point of view may themselves be taken as reflecting the inexorable linkage of pain and individuality. It is indicative that at the end of a remarkably comprehensive survey of the scientific literature on pain, a survey in which material drawn from 687 references has been discussed, the author laconically concludes, "Pain cannot be satisfactorily defined, except as every man defines it introspectively for himself."[2]

[1] O. Rank, *The trauma of birth* (New York: Harcourt, Brace, 1929).

[2] H. K. Beecher, "The measurement of pain," *Pharmacological Reviews* 9 (1957): 190.

Pain and the Functions of the Ego

In methodological discussions in which the ground of acceptable observation of psychological phenomena has come under examination, pain usually has a central place. Thus, for example, on September 6, 1965, there was a debate between Professor Brand Blanshard of the Philosophy Department at Yale University, and Professor B. F. Skinner of the Psychology Department at Harvard University at a convention of the American Psychological Association. The largest available hall was used. There was record attendance. The issue was "The problem of consciousness," essentially revolving around the admissibility to scientific scrutiny of experiences not evident in overt behavior. Pain, of course, became a central point of discussion. Professor Blanshard, criticizing Professor Skinner and the behaviorist position, argued:

> The most obvious [difficulty of the behaviorist position] is that the experience of pain, for example, is self-evidently not the same thing as a physical movement of any kind. . . . their identification is a confusion [that] can be shown in various ways. . . . If a pain were any kind of physical motion, we could ask what its direction and velocity were, whereas it makes no sense to talk of the direction and velocity of a toothache. On the other hand, we speak of pain as dull or excruciating, while a dull or excruciating motion is meaningless again.

Furthermore, Professor Blanshard pointed out, the behaviorist refutes his own position by his behavior, say, in the dentist's office, where he behaves in a way which can only make sense on the assumption that the behaviorist himself has accepted the reality of pain and decided that it is something to be averted. Skinner replied that the "two adjectives [dull and excruciating] are applied because they apply to things which cause

60

pain. A dull pain is the kind of pain caused by a dull object, as a sharp pain is caused by a sharp object. The term 'excruciating' is taken from the practice of crucifixion." And so the argument went.[3]

The problem inheres in the fact that pain is "private." If one insists that the data of psychology shall be "public," then pain has to be ruled out as being beyond the enclosing limit. Pain is ultimately private in that it is lodged in the individual person, the person individuated in many relevant respects out of the larger telos. If we insist that science be guided by a canon of what the contemporary philosophy of science jargon refers to as publicity, there simply cannot be a science of pain which can do justice to the phenomenon. Thus it turns out, paradoxically, as almost always the case with things connected with pain, that a methodological canon of science which is highly conditioned by man's social nature forces one into the position of essentially denying the existence of pain in the contexts in which it occurs.

We cannot accept this canon of method if we are to make progress. Although its existence is conditioned by the sense of the social telos, by the recognition of the necessity of some unity among the members of the scientific community at the very least, I believe that it is misguided. Like so many other human mechanisms, it has the appearance of serving that which it is, in point of fact, working to defeat. Also, although pain is essentially lonely, another paradox is that a cry of pain coming from one person may, at the very least, evoke in another an effort to help the person who is in pain; and thus pain is also a means of returning to the dominion of the social telos. For purposes of our discussion, let us

---

[3] I am indebted to Professor Blanshard for providing me with copies of both his and Professor Skinner's remarks.

admit and in no way minimize the reality or significance of pain in the total life of man.

The so-called stimulus-response psychologists are among the most scientifically self-conscious and scientifically meticulous. Yet, if we attempt to comprehend the phenomenon of pain from a scientific point of view, the stimulus-response point of view serves only to impede our progress. The stimulus-response psychologists would attempt to explain all psychological phenomena in terms of the relationships between characteristics of the stimuli and characteristics of the response. These psychologists typically understand stimulus as something external to the body, located in the environment but "impinging" on the body. The very distinction between stimulus and response, however, presumes a sharp, definitive distinction between the organism and the environment. In connection with pain, we are at the margin between stimulus and response, right *in* the organism. The attempt to classify pain as either stimulus or response is immediately handicapped and handicapping. For example, we run into difficulties at once from the stimulus-response point of view when we consider a paper with the title "Release of intracellular potassium as the physiological stimulus for pain."[4] Suppose that the author is correct in his belief that pain is experienced only when there is a release of intracellular potassium. Is it really correct to talk about the release of potassium as a stimulus? Is not the release of intracellular potassium equally a response? I do not wish to discuss the technical character of the relevant observations but only to make clear that the distinction between stimulus and response is based on a rather clear-cut distinction between organism and environment and that it is often

[4] F. B. Benjamin in *Journal of Applied Physiology* 14 (1959): 643–46.

precisely in those instances in which the neatness of division of organism and environment breaks down that we have pain. Aristotle perhaps rightly did not include pain among the senses.[5] Spinoza considered pain as an emotion.[6] With the emergence of modern physiology and physiological psychology, however, there has been an ongoing effort to categorize pain among the senses. From at least the time of Goldscheider[7] there have been efforts to identify pain receptors in the body, analogous to receptors for the other sense modalities. To this day research has not yielded definitive results; no anatomic proof for such specificity has been demonstrated. In the eighteenth century Erasmus Darwin put forth the notion that pain was the consequence of any excessive stimulation,[8] and in the twentieth century one very competent reviewer of the literature is brought to the conclusion that "pain may arise from virtually *any* type of stimulus or may be the result of afferent patterns which may travel via *any* available pathway."[9] The discovery of specific receptors would provide validation for considering pain along with the other senses and allow the possibility of conceptualizing it in purely stimu-

[5] *Nicomachean Ethics*, trans. D. Ross (London: Oxford University Press, 1954), Book II.

[6] B. de Spinoza, *The philosophy of Spinoza* (New York: Carlton House, 1927), p. 217.

[7] A. Goldscheider, "Die specifischen Functionen der Nerven der Haut," *Congrès Périodique International des Sciences Médicales* (Copenhagen, 1884), pp. 25–27, and "Die spezifische Energie der Gefühlsnerven der Haut," *Monatshefte für praktische Dermatologie* 3 (1884): 283–303.

[8] *Zoonomia, or, the laws of organic life* (London: J. Johnson, 1794), 1: 121, 125.

[9] W. Noordenbos, *Pain: problems pertaining to the transmission of nerve impulses which give rise to pain* (New York: Elsevier Publishing Co., 1959), p. 176.

lus-response terms. Unfortunately for the position of the stimulus-response psychologists, the data simply do not permit it.

A person in pain might try to tell someone else of the nature of his pain by saying, for example, that it is a "dull" pain, meaning that it is like the pain experienced when a dull object is pressed against the tissues. In attempting to explain the nature of pain one may borrow language associated with the other sense modalities. But the actual experience of pain is utterly lonely, without words of its own to describe it. One may attempt to reach out of the loneliness in some way, to describe it as "dull" or "sharp," or to take it as in some way connected with the redemption of mankind. But it remains true, as Beecher said, that "pain cannot be satisfactorily defined, except as every man defines it introspectively for himself." Pain is the burden of the organism separated out of the larger telos, and it is indicative of the decentralization of the individual telos of the organism. It is the ultimate of individual experience, expressible basically not in terms descriptive of the characteristics of objects such as "dull" and "sharp" but in those sounds one is able to make before learning to speak, especially the sound uttered at birth, the occasion when one is ripped from union into a condition of physical individuality.

The comment I have quoted from Skinner on the dull pain caused by a dull object, the sharp pain caused by a sharp object, and the excruciating pain caused, for example, by being nailed to a cross provides us with a hint of a way by which we can deepen our understanding of the nature of pain. He is, I believe, quite wrong. But the path into this error is itself instructive. Basic to Professor Skinner's position is the rather common notion that the skin is the boundary of the individual, that which takes place inside the envelope of skin being "within" the individual and that which takes place outside the envelope being "outside" of him. The normal, non-psychotic person in our culture characteristically thinks of himself this way. In other words, the normal person in our society develops an ego boundary which more or less coincides with the physical body as bounded by the skin; and so does a normal psychologist whose position in psychology is founded on such common sense.

A concept useful in understanding the nature of pain is distality. Distality may be defined as the *phenomenal distance* between an event or an object and "me," or simply "how far away from me" something appears to be. Although there are often substantial correlations between the physical distance from a part of the body to an external body and the phenomenal distance, the phenomenal distance and the physical distance are not necessarily the same. Egon Brunswik, from whom I am borrowing the term distality, considered the problem of ascertaining the precise way in which distality is related to the physical world as one of the most essential problems of psychology. The order of magnitude for the distalities of the different sense modalities varies considerably. We see things which are from a few inches to miles away. We hear sounds at various distances, but not so far as we can see. And we touch things which are, of course, no distance at all from us. The sense organs are important to the individual in that they inform him of the world "outside himself"; and distality is thus "how far outside" things are.

But consider the distality associated with pain. If we were to rank the sense modalities in accordance with the distality characteristic of each of them, and if we considered pain to be a sense modality, then clearly vision would be at the head of the list and pain at the other extreme, after touch. If the distality associated with touch is something slightly greater than zero, *the distality of pain is less than zero*.

A corollary to its negative distality is the fact that pain differs from the other sense modalities in being considerably less informative of the external world. It does not tell anything at all about that world's nature. The information contributed by pain is location within the body (and that being is in question, which will be discussed presently).

The blindness, as it were, of pain to the external world is another aspect of its utter association with the single individual. Skinner has a profound intuition, that what is social and public is made possible by the sharing of experiences conditioned by the stability of the external world. But unfortunately pain is so thoroughly associated with the individuality of the organism that Skinner must either abandon pain from his scientific purview or distort it, ascribing to it a distality like that of the other sense modalities, as essentially he does.

As I have said, pain demands interpretation. It demands interpretation partly because it is blind in this sense, blind to the external world. And, as I have also said, it is difficult to describe, if it can be described at all. Patients may speak of a "stabbing" or a "drawing" pain. But these are words or projections which attempt to identify the cause of the pain. Skinner also commits the classical "stimulus error," identified by Titchener, of attributing to the sensation the characteristics of the stimulus.[10] It may be pointed out parenthetically that the forms of psychology which stressed the significance of sensation, very largely out of British empiricism, went hand in hand with an intense individualism. Har-

[10] See E. G. Boring, *A history of experimental psychology*, 2d ed. (New York: Appleton-Century-Crofts, 1950), pp. 417 ff.

dy, Wolff, and Goodell devote the whole first chapter of their treatise on pain to the argument that pain is a sensation and not a feeling, although there is considerable irony in their having to admit that "recent evidence supports the old view that the feeling state may perchance be the most relevant aspect of pain to the one who suffers."[11] Skinner attributes dullness and the like—characteristics with distality drawn from other sense modalities—to pain. In this way he gives meaning to pain. One of the major roles of modern medicine is to give meaning to pain by discovering the forms of tissue injury which have led to a particular pain. The mother who has experienced the pain of childbirth finds its meaning in the relationship to the child whom she will care for, and who will announce his pain to her by crying out as she did so recently. Skinner is eminently correct in pointing out the great significance of the cross as a symbol of the meaning of pain, a symbol through which large segments of humanity could be joined together. For many centuries the cross has been the way in which many people have found meaning in pain. The cross and its context of meaning has pointed the way for them to a union with the cosmic, on the one hand, and humanity, on the other. Indeed, one might well argue that one of the major psychological uses of Christianity has been to overcome the essential loneliness and privacy of pain.

The Paradox of the Function of Pain

Paradox haunts just about every effort that has been made to understand the nature of pain. After reviewing

[11] J. D. Hardy, H. G. Wolff, and Helen Goodell, *Pain sensations and reactions* (Baltimore: Williams & Wilkins, 1952), p. 24.

the experimental facts on pain, Beecher said laconically, "Hardly an item has been mentioned for which there have not been opposing data to be considered."[12]

Among the many paradoxes associated with pain, one of the most significant is that pain seems to have both positive and negative values with respect to the continuing functioning of the organism and its survival. Thus, we find *both* the following statements, which are true yet in some way inconsistent with each other, in a major published treatise on pain. In one place we find:

> Pain, in its final analysis, is a warning signal against potential or actual damage to tissue cells. . . .[13]

In another place:

> As Leriche . . . pointed out, the idea that pain is always a beneficent mechanism constitutes "an extraordinary error, which has no justification." Under conditions where it becomes nagging and persistent, pain impairs the sufferer's ability to work and to think clearly, prevents his sleep, abolishes appetite, lowers morale, and may even destroy his will to help himself survive.[14]

I believe, however, that the resolution of the paradox is implicit in some of the considerations I have already advanced. In the chapter on disease I offered a number of considerations indicating that telic decentralization results, on the one hand, in organismic growth and development, and, on the other, in disease and death. In

---

[12] "The measurement of pain," p. 189.

[13] J. C. White and W. H. Sweet, *Pain: its mechanisms and neurosurgical control* (Springfield, Ill.: Charles C Thomas, 1955), p. 68.

[14] *Ibid.*, p. 99.

this chapter I have indicated that we are to regard pain as the manifestation of telic decentralization. Thus, pain is similarly associated with individual survival, on the one hand, and disease and death, on the other.

Pain as the psychic manifestation of telic decentralization is not merely epiphenomenal to telic decentralization. It is rather an extremely important factor in the whole process of telic decentralization. There can be little question about the individual-survival-positive character of pain. Sometimes, as the Darwinian type of thinking has led us to observe, pain is a signal that telic decentralization is taking place, and pain may provoke the processes whereby the larger telos takes over and stops the decentralization. Pain produces the outcry which evokes help by others. The sounds caused by pain which are made by infants and even adults are part of the universal language of man, transcending all cultural differences, and have the singular meaning of "Help!" Cries of pain lead to nursing (in both senses of the word, suckle and care for) responses on the part of others. Pain is characteristically inversely related to well-being; and very often (though, not always) the increase or decrease of pain indicates whether one is hindering or aiding the survival and well-being of the individual. An injury to a particular part of the body usually leads to a rather drastic lowering of the pain threshold in that part. This increase in pain-sensitivity leads the individual to act in such a way as to protect and spare that particular part of the body, giving it time to heal. Pain also encourages a decrease in motility of the individual which is conducive to recovery. Pain is associated, too, with learning; the experience of pain in a given situation teaches the individual to avoid that situation in the future. Pain thus tends to increase the chances of survival, since that which gives pain may, unchecked, lead to death. Pain may even be a spur to success. George Engel has reported the case of a man who suffered intense pain and yet was extremely successful in his work. When measures were found by which to eliminate the pain, the man no longer performed successfully.[15]

Nor can there be any doubt that pain can equally be individual-survival-negative. In its overwhelming demands for the attention of the ego, it can thoroughly incapacitate the individual. Thus both of the quotations cited above are true in spite of the discrepancy between them.

Pain as a Demand upon a Higher Telos

One of the most interesting paradoxes associated with pain is that it may be considered as either purely physical or purely psychological. On the one hand, pain is clearly a phenomenon associated with the physical body. The person in pain can usually indicate its location, sometimes with inordinate specificity. If asked whether the pain is physical or psychological, he will reply that it is physical. The idea that pain is a psychological condition can make little sense to the person experiencing it.

And yet, on the other hand, with a slight shift in perspective, it is also quite clear that pain is psychological. In a banal but logical sense, unless there is a psyche, unless there is an awake and conscious organism, there is nothing to which one can sensibly refer as pain. Pain exists only in a conscious ego. If it is pain, then it is not unconscious. Drugs that influence pain, such as alcohol, ether, and barbiturates, also have the effect of modify-

[15] G. L. Engel, "Guilt, pain, and success," *Psychosomatic Medicine* 24 (1962): 37–48.

ing the ego functions or suspending them altogether by putting the individual to sleep. Stimulation of the ego functions by other means, such as the presentation of intense auditory stimulation, may reduce or abolish pain.[16] Exercises in the direction of attention, such as those practiced by yogis, seem to cancel pain. Radical surgery has been performed on people under hypnosis without signs of pain. Prize fighters, football players, soldiers in battle, and others engaged in activities demanding intense concentration may show no signs of pain even when severely injured.

It has been pointed out that there is a great discrepancy between the progress that has been made in the alleviation of pain and the progress that has been made in unraveling the mysteries of the pain phenomenon itself.[17] This discrepancy is not really so hard to understand, since so much of the alleviation of pain is achieved simply by the use of drugs. We need not understand the mechanisms whereby these drugs affect the ego functions to be able to use them in the management of pain.

Pain, having no other locus but the conscious ego, is almost literally the price man pays for the possession of a conscious ego, as the biblical story of Adam and Eve in the Garden of Eden so strongly suggests: Eve, having eaten of the Tree of Knowledge, must bear her children in pain. There is some reason to believe that the higher up in the evolutionary scale the organism is, the more likely that organism is to possess anything that can be identified as pain. It has even been suggested that observed group differences in pain thresholds may be ex-

[16] See W. J. Gardner, J. C. R. Licklider, and A. Z. Weisz, "Suppression of pain by sound," *Science* 132 (1960): 32.

[17] J. J. Bonica, *The management of pain* (Philadelphia: Lea & Febiger, 1953), p. 22.

plained in terms of different degrees of development of consciousness among groups.[18] Certainly the most effective devices available for the elimination of pain are exactly those which eliminate consciousness entirely.

A certain degree of psychological development is a prerequisite for being able to experience pain. Puppies raised under conditions of stimulus deprivation, which has been demonstrated to have the effect of keeping animals from developing psychologically,[19] show no pain reaction even when subject to flame and pin pricks.[20]

In the preceding chapter I indicated that disease may be understood as the separation of lower telê from higher telê in the organism and suggested that the conscious ego might be understood as the major telic center of the organism. Pain, I have said, is the manifestation of telic decentralization. Let me now add the consideration that pain is the demand on the conscious ego to work to bring the decentralized part back into the unity of the organism. Pain is the imperative to the ego to assume the responsibility of telic centralization, the ego itself having emerged as a result of telic decentralization. Let us return for a moment to the consideration of the example of the boil or abscess cited by Selye. According to Selye there is a disproportionate response to injury and it is this very response that makes for the inflammation. In addition, however, the person with the inflammation is also experiencing pain, which is a demand on the part of

[18] *Ibid.*, p. 83.

[19] A. H. Riesen, "Stimulation as a requirement for growth and function in behavioral development," in D. Fiske and S. R. Maddi, eds., *Functions of varied experience* (Homewood, Ill.: Dorsey Press, 1961), pp. 57–80.

[20] R. Melzack and T. H. Scott, "The effects of early experience on the response to pain," *Journal of Comparative and Physiological Psychology* 50 (1957): 155–61.

the locus of inflammation for attention from the ego. The ego must act to reduce the inflammation, or the pain will continue. Thus the healing arts may be viewed as a collective result of man's ego's efforts to overcome the telic decentralization announced by pain.

The Phenomenally Ego-Alien Nature of Pain

Both the formation of the ego and the development of the capacity for experiencing pain itself in the life of an individual organism are the result of telic decentralization. But the organism, in a certain sense having created pain, reacts by being averse to it. Pain then becomes a means to the further decentralization of the telos. One of the major ways by which the decentralization takes place is in pain's appearing to the ego as being alien to it.

Again, paradoxically, pain is both psychologically determined and phenomenally ego-alien. The literature is replete with examples, from both before and after 1895 when Breuer and Freud's study of hysteria appeared,[21] which provide clear-cut evidence that psychological processes play a determinative role in the generation of pain. The ego can bring about experiences which are alien to itself. As but one example, an investigator found that he could induce pain in the phantom limbs of nine out of twenty-two amputees

> by referring to some cause of anxiety in the patient's interpersonal life. For instance, although one patient complained of persistent pain, it was noted that he was without discomfort throughout

[21] J. Breuer and S. Freud, *Studien über Hysterie* (Leipzig: F. Deuticke, 1895).

the diagnostic interview, except when certain emotionally charged subjects were discussed. These were: the possible reaction of his wife to the disfigurement, his fear that she might leave him and, less noticeably, his mother's illness. When these topics were introduced into the discussion, the patient grasped the amputation stump, jerked his head toward the right shoulder and then complained of having pain. This psychologic evocation of pain occurred repeatedly; the introduction of these topics, psychologically painful to him, led him to behave in this manner.[22]

Phenomenally, however, pain appears to the conscious ego as not a part of itself, but as alien to it, as something happening *to* the ego, with the ego, as it were, the victim of external forces. Here we have a significant difference between what we may judge analytically to be the fact and the phenomenology of the case. On the one hand, our judgment, informed by numerous evidences, exemplified by Kolb's report on amputees, indicates that pain may be generated psychologically, albeit unconsciously. On the other hand, the normal ego processes characteristically would cause the pain to be experienced as quite alien to the psyche. The phenomenally ego-alien quality of pain is indicated by White and Sweet in the following manner:

> In patients we have studied the pain has almost universally been described as "it," an objectified stimulus which causes varying degrees of stress. On the whole the patient related this stimulus to

[22] L. C. Kolb, *The painful phantom: psychology, physiology and treatment* (Springfield, Ill.: Charles C Thomas, 1954), p. 21.

the "I" by describing "it" as present in a certain part of the body.[23]

Let us pause here to consider a somewhat parenthetical, yet significant point, to which I have alluded earlier. There are normal ego processes which themselves interfere with the appreciation of the nature of human suffering. Such a possibility was indicated by Freud's observation that the mechanisms of repression and resistance by their very nature not only play their role in neuroses but also are involved in an individual's difficulty in appreciating the contributions of psychoanalysis itself. The field of psychosomatic medicine has long suffered from the handicap of the ego's externalizing the source of its suffering. There is a genuine aversion to the notion that pain may be in any way psychologically induced. We can understand this aversion. As the epigraph has it, "When I thought to know this, it was too painful for me." To conceive of pain as the product of psychological processes, rather than as something done to the psyche, appears to undermine the very work of the ego in its attempt to manage the pain, that is, to convert pain to an ego-alien status. The deeper truth is, of course, that in so doing the ego is engaging in exactly the process which is associated with pain in the first place. Freud's observation that the same repression which is associated with not accepting the contributions of psychoanalysis is at work in forming the neurosis is a special instance of a much more general phenomenon.

As I have indicated, in ordinary circumstances the boundary of the ego is more or less coincident with the boundary of the body. The ego is, as Freud put it, "first and foremost a body-ego." "I" and "me" are hardly dissociated from the body. They are phenomenally one,

[23] *Pain*, p. 108.

as contrasted with the remainder of the environment, which is "other." Pain has its role in the decentralization which the distinction between "I" and other represents, and in the creation of the identification of the ego with the boundary of the body. This very decentralization probably involves the identification of "what hurts me" as something external to the ego, with the body thus remaining internal to it, or at least coinciding with it.

As the ego develops, a differentiated view of the body normally takes place in which again pain plays a significant role; for one of the important characteristics of pain is, as has already been indicated, its localization in the body. *The ego, in managing pain, seeks to make pain distal with respect to the ego itself*, if it cannot make it distal with respect to the body. As the ego develops, the question of where the injury is becomes extremely significant. But it is in this process that pain gets differentiated into the " 'it' as present in a certain part of the body," with the body itself becoming something "other" to the ego.

There are obvious benefits associated with the fact that pain is phenomenally ego-alien. By placing the affected part of the body in the outside world, as it were, the ego provides itself with the psychological precondition for engaging in such efforts as may be needed for reducing further damage and repairing injury, such as withdrawing the affected part from the noxious condition, extracting the thorn from the skin, applying medical measures to the affected part, or directing the attention of those who would help to the part of the body which needs attention. In other words, the ego-alien pain provides "information" whereby the ego may act in a way consonant with the telos of the total organ-

76

ism, repairing the affected part and restoring it into the whole.

At the same time, however, the affected part of the body becomes "other" to the ego, and as such allows the ego to surrender that part of the body which is already partially separated telically from the rest of the body. The tooth in which there is pain becomes "the tooth that hurts me," an "it" which is no longer "me"; and its extraction is not an injury to the ego but a saving of the ego from assault. This psychological process of turning a part of "me" into "it" is thus preparatory for actually getting rid of it. Getting rid of pain often means getting rid of the affected part. This dynamic associated with the ego's processes was magnificently rendered in the Sermon on the Mount: "And if thy right eye offend thee, pluck it out. . . . And if thy right hand offend thee, cut it off, and cast it from thee: for it is profitable for thee that one of thy members should perish, and not that thy whole body should be cast into hell" (Matt. 5:29–30). And perhaps the very pain of childbirth is functionally linked to getting rid of that which is causing the pain, so as to produce the new separated being, the child.

To summarize, in the normal instance there are two functions performed by making pain ego-alien: one, providing a psychological precondition for engaging in acts of rectification; and, two, preparing to sacrifice the affected part. But these are clearly in conflict.

By virtue of the conflict thus engendered, agony is added to pain. The ego is presented with a conflict, and this conflict reflects the telic decentralization within the ego itself. For, on the one hand, pain is a demand upon the ego to overcome the telic decentralization which the pain is signaling. On the other hand, pain suggests that the affected part should be completely separated from the rest of the organism. The conflict which may be involved in deciding whether or not to amputate an arm or a leg is a paradigmatic conflict of the ego in its experience of pain. The agony is compounded by the fact that in both instances there is a threat to the very life of the individual, bringing his being into question. Pain in any part of the organism contains within it the threat of death, which I shall discuss later in some detail. At the same time something like the loss of a limb constitutes the literal death of at least a part which was once integral to the ego. Pain is a harbinger of death beyond all the options associated with its management.

The fact of the matter is that the continued existence of the organism and its ego is contingent upon the continued existence of the body. In some instances one might even opt, consciously or unconsciously, for continued pain rather than the complete "it-izing"—if a neologism be permitted—of a part. Some of the observers of amputees with pain in a phantom limb have sought to comprehend the nature of these cases as being that the patient has *not* succeeded in fully converting the missing limb to an "it," still conceiving of the limb as "me." As Kolb puts it, "The occurrence of the phantom is best explained as the patient's enduring concept of his total body image after the loss of a part through amputation."[24] In many instances patients who have lost limbs through surgery manifest inordinate, and even pathological, interest in the amputated limb. Szasz has suggested that the psychodynamic processes of pain in the phantom limb have the unconscious meaning to the patient that "that part hurts and is therefore present."[25]

[24] *The painful phantom*, p. 8.

[25] T. S. Szasz, *Pain and pleasure: a study of bodily feelings* (New York: Basic Books, 1957), p. 162.

The Pain-Annihilation Complex

It is too much to say that a cell in the condition just prior to cellular fission is in pain. There is little evidence that anything like consciousness exists in the cell; there is certainly nothing to indicate that it makes any sense at all to talk of the ego of a cell; and there is nothing to indicate that a cell about to divide into two separated cells experiences a sense that it, as an individual, is about to be annihilated. Nonetheless, it is helpful to think of the processes which precede the fundamental form of telic decentralization, cellular fission, as formally the same as those which, in the higher organism endowed with consciousness, make for pain. Our thought is led to that normal condition of pain, the pain of parturition, in which that single telic unit, the mother and the fetus, must divide into two organisms. And our thought is brought to the idea of sacrifice in which that which is "me" is made into something which is "not-me," and in which that "not-me" is sacrificed in order that "I" might continue to live. The sacrifice of an affected limb is of essentially the same order psychologically as the sacrifice of the child, a matter to be dealt with in the next chapter. In both instances of sacrifice the pain which precedes it is indicative of the basic underlying telic decentralization. But let us hold off our discussion of sacrifice and consider here what we may call the *pain-annihilation complex*.

The idea that I have been developing here is that pain is indicative of telic decentralization. In the previous chapter it was indicated that telic decentralization leads eventually to disease and death. Pain is then, also, indicative of the fact that death will eventually ensue. The matter is, of course, complicated by the fact that telic decentralization is also associated with positive growth and development. Therefore, the conscious ego sensibly asks in each instance whether the particular pain it is experiencing is one of those pains which is indicative of the particular stage of telic decentralization that leads quickly into death. Each pain provokes the question, Does this pain mean that I will die? The possibility of annihilation is then necessarily a component of the psychological processes associated with the experience of pain.

One of the important characteristics of the ego is that it is aware of the possibility of its own annihilation. To put it this way, however, is to presuppose a certain high level of development of the ego. In the early stages of ego development, there is rather a primitive pain-annihilation complex in which pain and the sense of the possibility of annihilation are not yet separated. We may, in our own more mature and sophisticated stage of ego development, analyze the primitive pain experience into the two components of pain per se and annihilation. But primitively the ego experiences pain as an undifferentiated "I-am-being-hurt-and-killed." The very separation of the sense of annihilation from pain per se is itself an instance of telic decentralization. Yet it is instructive to recognize these two components in the total phenomenological complex.

In the normal maturation of the ego, these two components of the pain experience may become differentiated. The organism may experience pain per se without at the same time experiencing a sense of being annihilated or, for that matter, may experience a sense of being annihilated without experiencing pain per se. At this point we need to recall the earlier discussion on the tendency to distalize pain. In the differentiation of pain per se from the sense of being annihilated, pain per se is localized as outside the ego, whereas the sense of being annihilated is retained inside the ego. Thus it is only pain per se which is made ego-alien. The differentiated sense of being annihilated is what is commonly referred to as *anxiety*, and may be further identified with what Heidegger has termed "being at issue."[26] I do not mean to give the impression that I believe all anxiety to be based in some initial experience involving pain per se. There is, as has been pointed out by Kessen and Mandler, substantial evidence that anxiety can occur without pain, in response, for example, to frustration, interruption of activities, the appearance of a stranger to a young child, and a loud noise. Anxiety also occurs among persons who are congenitally analgesic.[27] The mature person, say, who readily submits to an inoculation is one in whom the distinction is firmly drawn. His ego is fully aware that his being is not at issue, that he is not being annihilated, and that the pain is nothing but pain per se. A child in the doctor's office who "cries as though he were being killed" has probably not differentiated the sense of annihilation from pain per se.

The ego, however, experiences a major difficulty in fully separating pain per se from the sense of being annihilated. The "reality principle" enters. For, in point of fact, the continued existence of the ego *is* contingent upon the continued existence of the body; and tissue injury *is* indicative of the possibility of annihilation. Thus, characteristically the ego actually believes, as

[26] M. Heidegger, *Being and Time*, trans. J. Macquarrie and E. Robinson (New York: Harper & Row, 1962), pp. 67 ff. I am indebted to my wife, Dr. Mildred Bakan, for help in appreciating the relevance of this notion for the phenomenon of pain, and especially for the particular context of meaning that she placed upon it in "On self-consciousness," *Existential Psychiatry* (1969), 7, pp. 43–60.

[27] W. Kessen and G. Mandler, "Anxiety, pain, and the inhibition of distress," *Psychological Review* 68 (1961): 396–404.

some research workers have asserted, that the "adequate stimulus" for pain is tissue damage. "Tissue damage, then, often extremely slight and completely reversible, becomes the keystone of the type of adjustments, sensations, feeling states, and behavior that constitute the pain experience."[28] Any approach to the problem of pain cannot overlook this fact, which every normal person "knows." We, however, must understand this on two levels. The first is the common sense level, the normal one, that tissue injury causes pain. The second is that the ego characteristically believes this. It is this very belief on the part of the ego which prevents the total psychological dissociation of pain per se from the sense of annihilation. An important element connected with the tenaciousness of the ego in holding to this belief is the corresponding belief that there is a relationship between the extent of tissue injury and the intensity of pain: the more intense the pain, the greater the injury, and the greater the threat to being. If we consider the evidence, however, the fact is that tissue injury in the simple sense in which the ego holds it cannot be considered the "cause" of pain. It fails as a cause by the simple application of the principle: if A is the cause of B, then we should get B if and only if A is present. Tissue injury is not an adequate explanation of pain. There are instances in which there is pain without tissue injury, and instances in which there is tissue injury without pain.

When the ego has to some degree differentiated the sense of annihilation from pain per se, and when the sense of annihilation has been aroused, as it can be for many reasons other than tissue injury, the ego mechanisms, unconscious though they may be, may function

[28] Hardy, Wolff, and Goodell, *Pain sensations and reactions*, p. 379.

to encourage pain per se in order to make it possible for the ego to act upon the "cause," the presumptive tissue injury, and thus reduce the sense of annihilation. The very belief that tissue injury is the cause of pain, which has some basis in fact, may be entailed in the generation of pain per se itself, as in the case of Kolb's amputees. If we consider pain as the manifestation of telic decentralization and anxiety as the sense of being annihilated, or, to use the existentialist term, the sense of one's "being at issue," then the "conversion" of the sense of being annihilated to pain at least has the appearance of giving one a chance to live, as it were, since there is the promise implicit in pain that the ego may do something to avert death. Unfortunately, sometimes this "conversion" does not help, and one has further pain for one's unconscious psychological trouble.

What I have said here indicates a possible explanation for what is certainly one of the greatest puzzles associated with pain, masochistic behavior. I suggest that the person who engages in masochistic behavior is one in whom the sense of annihilation and pain per se are relatively strongly differentiated and in whom, furthermore, the sense of possible annihilation itself is strong. In masochistic behavior, inflicting pain upon oneself is an effort to rebind the sense of annihilation to pain per se, thus affording the ego the sense of control over sources of annihilation.

An essential feature of an organism which can experience pain is that it is multicellular and multi-organed, and that the organism can survive as an individual in spite of some loss of tissue. The possibility of splitting the sense of annihilation from pain per se derives chiefly from the fact that pain is highly, and even quite precisely, localized, especially in those parts of the body which can be surrendered with less likelihood of annihilation. Indeed, the localization of pain where there is injury to a vital internal organ is generally considerably less precise, often demonstrating, for example, the phenomenon of "referred pain," in which pain is ascribed to a locus quite different from that of any actual tissue injury. When a vital internal organ suffers injury, life itself is critically at issue, and the possibility of differentiating the sense of annihilation from pain per se is diminished. Differentiation is more easily achieved if the individual can survive with loss of the affected tissue. Then the ego can withdraw from the injured part, allowing the phenomenally alien pain per se but reserving survival to the ego itself, and to those parts upon which the continued existence of the body is still contingent.

We are now in a position to throw some light on the question of psyche and soma, the question which confounds so much of the thought and research in connection with disease. Pain is, as it were, its touchstone, since pain is so intimately related to both psyche and soma. The resolution of the question is in the recognition that the very creation of the conscious ego is the result of the process of telic decentralization, with the central telos of the organism being chiefly lodged in the conscious ego, a specialization of the total telos of the organism itself. One of the major instrumentalities of the ego's effectiveness is that which leads the ego to separate itself from the body to which it ascribes pain. Through the instrumentality of pain, therefore, the central telos of the organism itself is subject to further telic decentralization.

The ego separates itself from the soma; and thus the soma loses the telic centralization function of the ego itself. But as we have seen, especially in the discussion of Selye's research, it is precisely telic decentralization which is associated with the generation of many diseases. This, of course, leads to further pain which the ego would again avert by locating the pain outside of the ego in the body, depriving the body of the function of the ego as telic centralizer, and so on, until death ensues.

Thus, it appears that the ego needs pain in order to function. Yet its very functioning involves the attempt to rid itself of pain. The ego, itself the result of telic decentralization, functions by telic decentralization as well as by telic centralization. Realizing its incarnateness, it aims to preserve itself *and* the body but at the same time tends to separate itself from the body. While it is "first and foremost a body-ego," its emergence is the product of the same process, telic decentralization which will ultimately lead to the destruction of the body. Finally, by seeking to withdraw itself from the body, the ego seeks also to save itself from annihilation; yet this very withdrawal is itself a factor in its annihilation.

Some Empirical Studies

There are some data available which point to the ego's ability and tendency to differentiate between the sense of annihilation, phenomenally reserved inside the ego, and pain per se as localized in the body and distal with respect to the ego.

A characteristic remark often made by patients who have been treated for pain by barbiturates or morphine, or who have undergone prefrontal lobotomy, is, "My pain is the same, but it doesn't hurt me now."[29] Such a remark indicates that these medical measures somehow result in the separation of the sense of annihilation from pain per se and in a reduction of the sense of annihilation. A series of related studies[30] on the effects of morphine indicates that morphine acts not to reduce the pain thresholds as such, since the pain thresholds to experimentally induced pain were not changed, but rather to reduce the anxiety, what we are calling the sense of being annihilated, or the sense of "being at issue."

A study by Petrie suggests that one of the effects of prefrontal lobotomy is to increase the distality of touch and kinesthesis, and it may increase the distality of pain per se as well. It has been found that after a prefrontal lobotomy the patient tends to judge the size of a handled block of wood as *smaller* than he did before the lobotomy.[31] Although other interpretations are certainly possible, this finding can be considered indicative

[29] H. K. Beecher, "Pathology and experiment in advancing study of subjective responses, with emphasis on pain," in H. K. Beecher, ed., *Disease and the advancement of basic science* (Cambridge, Mass.: Harvard University Press, 1960), p. 228.

[30] H. E. Hill, C. H. Kornetsky, H. G. Flanary, and A. Wikler, "Effects of anxiety and morphine on discrimination intensities of painful stimuli," *Journal of Clinical Investigation* 31 (1952): 473–80, and "Studies on anxiety associated with anticipation of pain. I. Effects of morphine," *Archives of Neurology and Psychiatry* 67 (1952): 612–19; C. Kornetsky, "Effects of anxiety and morphine on the anticipation and perception of painful radiant thermal stimuli," *Journal of Comparative and Physiological Psychology* 47 (1954): 130–32; R. B. Malmo and C. Shagass, "Physiologic studies of reaction to stress in anxiety and early schizophrenia," *Psychosomatic Medicine* 11 (1949): 9–24, and "Physiologic study of symptom mechanisms in psychiatric patients under stress," *ibid.*, pp. 25–29.

[31] Asenath Petrie, "Some psychological aspects of pain and the relief of suffering," *Annals of the New York Academy of Sciences* 86 (1960): 13–27. See also Asenath Petrie, *Individuality in pain and suffering* (Chicago: University of Chicago Press, 1967).

of greater distality in general, the mechanism being analogous to the size-distance relationship in visual perception. The prefrontal lobotomy may have had the effect of increasing the distality of all perception.

Beecher compared manifestations of pain in wounded soldiers from the Anzio beachhead in World War II with those in civilians after surgery.[32] In response to questions about whether they wanted something to relieve their pain, only one-third of the soldiers answered affirmatively, compared to 80 per cent of the civilians. The explanation of this great discrepancy is, according to Beecher, in the meaning and significance of the wound. The men brought in from the Anzio beachhead had been living in great danger of being killed. Being wounded, and still being alive, being brought into the safety of the hospital, being aware that for them the war was over, had the effect of reducing the sense that they were about to be annihilated. Their wounded condition meant that the threat of annihilation was reduced. Among civilians, however, the total context associated with surgery, in contrast to other contexts of civilian life, itself suggests that death may be imminent.[33] Thus, according to our interpretation, which is consistent with that offered by Beecher, the discrepancy in the data between the two groups is explained by conceiving of a separation of the sense of annihilation from pain per se and a differential effect of the situations on the sense of annihilation. It may be objected that the amount of tissue trauma in the civilian situation may have been greater. Beecher

[32] H. K. Beecher, "Relationship of significance of wound to the pain experienced," *Journal of the American Medical Association* 161 (1956): 1609–13.

[33] See S. Bernstein and S. Small, "Psychodynamic factors in surgery," *Journal of Mt. Sinai Hospital* 17 (1951): 940–45, in which it is indicated that many patients envisage surgery itself as a death threat.

has indicated, however, that the amount of tissue trauma in the war situation was generally greater than that in the surgery situation. Thus, if extent of tissue trauma is in any way related to pain, pain per se may have been greater in the war situation. But the important difference was in the sense of annihilation.

At issue in the scientific study of pain is whether so-called experimental pain, pain induced in the laboratory, often with the investigators themselves as the subjects, leads to valid, or, at any rate, general conclusions. Beecher has been critical of such studies on the grounds that they do not duplicate the deep threat which is associated with real sickness or injury. He says, for example, "Not much imagination is needed to suppose that the sickbed of the patient in pain with its ominous threat against his happiness, his security, his very life, provides a milieu *and reaction* entirely different from the laboratory."[34] If human beings can split the sense of annihilation from pain per se, then we might expect that in the laboratory this split is readily made, for the very context of the laboratory is such that full provision is made that the pain will be *only* pain, and that the subject of the investigation will be under no threat of annihilation. Beecher comments laconically that among these investigators "anxiety must have become slight or non-existent."[35]

That human beings may vary in their ability to differentiate the sense of annihilation from pain per se is strongly indicated by the findings of two investigations. First, there is the observation by Hardy, Wolff, and Goodell that there is very little variation of pain

[34] "The measurement of pain," p. 168.

[35] *Ibid.*, p. 135.

thresholds among individuals.[36] The subjects they used in coming to this conclusion, however, were highly experienced in the laboratory. We can presume that one effect of the total laboratory milieu is precisely to facilitate the split of the sense of annihilation from pain per se, with the former being quite negligible. Second, there is the observation that substantial variation in pain thresholds exists among relatively naïve subjects, and substantial correlations among different types of thresholds over the group. In one study six different pain thresholds were determined for forty-six men who had volunteered for the Canadian army. Pain thresholds were determined for heat, electric shock, and pressure, and each again for pain-tolerance level.[37] The variation among individuals in this situation and with these subjects was considerably greater than that found by Hardy, Wolff, and Goodell. What is perhaps of equal or even greater significance is that the correlations among these six thresholds were quite substantial. If pain per se were being measured alone we should perhaps find little variation among the thresholds from individual to individual. But the further fact that the correlations ran relatively high indicates that there is an organismic factor operative in the determination of each of the six thresholds, and that this factor varies from individual to individual. Clark and Bindra, in discussing these data, argue that there is what they call an "affective" or "attitudinal" factor. I suggest that this attitudinal factor may perhaps be indicative of different degrees of differentiation of the sense of annihilation from pain per se, and varying degrees of arousal of the sense of annihilation, as one goes from subject to subject. Earlier I

[36] *Pain sensations and reactions.*

[37] J. W. Clark and D. Bindra, "Individual differences in pain thresholds," *Canadian Journal of Psychology* 10 (1956): 69–81.

suggested that the degree of telic decentralization is a characteristic of the total organism and that it varies from individual to individual. These data may be interpreted as bearing on that assertion—that perhaps the degree of telic decentralization is a characteristic of the total organism which is equally manifested in the degree of differentiation of pain per se from the sense of annihilation among the naïve subjects.

Placebos evidently succeed in reducing the amount of experienced pain in a certain proportion of cases. Beecher has reviewed fourteen studies involving twenty-six groups of patients in which the effect of placebos as pain relievers was studied.[38] The percentages in which relief was obtained varied from 15 to 58, the median being 35 per cent. Thus, over a wide range of studies, roughly a third of the persons in pain, given a placebo, experienced relief. Clearly it is hardly saline or lactose (or bicarbonate of soda in the case of angina pectoris) that brings relief, at least not by direct physiological action. We suggest that placebos work with patients in whom the differentiation of the sense of annihilation from the pain per se can readily be made and that in the total context in which the placebo is given the patient senses that he is being taken care of, that his "being" is not "at issue."

The considerations offered in this chapter hardly presume to be an exhaustive account of the nature of pain. Although there have been a few rather interesting recent attempts to understand the psychology of pain,[39] pain has resisted adequate conceptualization and requires

[38] "Pathology and experiment . . . ," p. 225.

[39] E.g., F. J. J. Buytendijk, *Pain*, trans. Eda O'Shiel (Chicago: University of Chicago Press, 1962; London: Hutchinson, 1961); Szasz, *Pain and pleasure*; Petrie, *Individuality in pain and suffering.*

extensive further thought and research. In the past few years a number of investigators have somehow succeeded in overcoming the great cultural resistance toward considering death an intellectual problem. Among these investigators have been the existentialist thinkers, for whom the question of "being" and "not-being" is taken as the central one. This presentation has to some degree been informed by such thought, for it is evident that pain is somehow very close to the question of being and not-being.

With its emergence as the manifestation of the central telos of the organism, the conscious ego acquired pain and purpose; and it sometimes purposes immortality. Pain and mortality make up the tragedy of man. Within these he squirms around. That conscious ego, however, is also capable of becoming identified with a larger telos of which the conscious ego is itself but a part. That larger telos appears to be immortal; and perhaps through its cultivation man can overcome the many subtragedies associated with the denial of his mortality. He need not sacrifice himself out of deference to the inexorable. Let him allow the inexorable to work itself out. Inexorability needs no help.

III

Sacrifice
and the
Book of Job

MY GOD, my GOD,
why hast thou forsaken me?
PSALM 22:1, MATT. 27:46, and MARK 15:34

BUT thou art he
that took me out of the womb:
thou didst make me hope
when I was upon my mother's breasts.
I was cast upon thee from the womb:
thou art my GOD
from my mother's belly.
BE not far from me;
for trouble is near;
for there is none to help.
PSALM 22:9–11

IN THIS chapter I shall attempt to engage in a more direct confrontation of the existential dimension in suffering than I have in the previous chapters. As a means to this end, I shall make use of the Bible, especially the Book of Job. The technical literature on pain often concedes that there are factors in connection with pain which cannot be encompassed by classical forms of neurology and physiology. Yet that literature only hints at the substance which is beyond. Indeed it could be argued —although I do not want to dwell here on this point— that the very problem of how to conceptualize pain involves the conflict between physical and existential views, the separation of views itself being an instance of the decentralization of the telos in members of the intellectual community. It is evident, however, considering our discussion of the clinical literature in the preceding chapter, that pain is simply too elusive to be grasped without taking the sense of annihilation into account. But the sense of annihilation is precisely the existentialist sense of being becoming non-being. In the discussion of the ego and its management of pain it became evident that there is an underlying process in which the ego tends to withdraw from the soma in preparation for its sacrifice. The biblical text provides an opportunity to consider sacrifice itself more fully.

I once heard a real cry of agony, unlike anything else I have ever heard. It was a lovely fall day in a crowded Jewish cemetery near New York City. A well-dressed middle-aged woman was on her knees embracing a tombstone and crying in Yiddish, "Papa, Papa, don't hit me! I beg you!" I have no way to reproduce the agony of that cry. It may have been that such a cry came from Jesus as he uttered words from the 22d Psalm, from which I have quoted above.

The Bible as a Psychological Document

I have thus far attempted to conceptualize the tragedy of man as a complex of pain, mortality, and consciousness. The line of thought leads to religion, to the realm of ultimate concern, to use Paul Tillich's term, and to the Bible as one of its major expressions. The Bible is an unusual book. There is no single set of texts which can match it in terms of influence on our civilization. Indeed the boundaries of what we may consider our civilization both in time and geography are determinable by what has or has not come under its influence. Although we are currently in a very secular stage, we must nonetheless recognize the fact that the Bible is a critical, if not the most critical, document, both affecting and expressing our culture. There must be something in man himself and in the Bible which makes the Bible appeal widely and deeply, generation after generation of men finding pertinence in it to their lives. It is not necessary to settle whether the Bible has formed the mind of Western man, or expresses something intrinsic in the mind of man. In either case we have a license to examine the Bible as a possible means for understanding man. Nonetheless, some disclaimers are in order.

The Bible as a Psychological Document

First, the divine character of the Bible need not be argued here. I presume to read the Bible as a psychological document.[1] This is not without precedent. Several modern thinkers, still within the Judeo-Christian tradition, have leaned toward an anthropocentric theology. I do not think that the Bible is degraded by reading it from such a perspective. Nor does it preclude other ways of reading it.

I do not know what divinity there is outside the compass of man's humanity. Indeed, to probe the question of why man should find it necessary or desirable to fashion divine images for himself in coping with his existential condition, a question which may be regarded as seditious in some theological contexts, is itself to advance our understanding of the nature of the divine.

Second, I do not presume to engage in biblical or literary criticism in the respective disciplinary senses, although some problems of canon and literary form are nonetheless relevant and will be discussed. The relevant discipline is psychology.

Third, even from the psychological point of view, I do not regard the biblical personages as "cases" in a clinical sense.

Fourth, certainly the Bible cannot be taken as an authoritative psychological text for any psychological assertions that I would like to make.

Rather, one might presume a kind of *biblical mind* which expressed itself in writing the Bible. Our interest is in seeking to understand the thought, feeling, and volition which this mind expressed. All that we have of the Bible is the text that lies before us. But one cannot

[1] See G. W. Allport, *The use of personal documents in psychological science* (New York: Social Science Research Council, 1942); J. Dollard, *Criteria for the life history* (New Haven: Yale University Press, 1935).

do justice to any text unless one supposes that it is the expression of a mind, and unless one seeks to understand the latter. The Bible, however, is not the product of one mind. It is the expression of many. Yet, those various minds which contributed to the Bible may be regarded as constituting a coherent whole in spite of all discrepancies. Every tradition has an organic unity over and beyond its individual contributors and participants. Each person within a tradition interacts with its past and is integrated into its future. It is reasonable to think of a tradition as constituting a single mentality (even with its conflicts and even with diverse influences upon it) without having to accept such obscurities as Jung's "collective unconscious" or the like.

The Canonical and Literary Character of the Book of Job

The Bible has a special characteristic which makes it important for us: it is canonical. It thus bespeaks the continuity and coherence of the whole of the relevant culture, not merely that of its authors. Indeed, the Bible arises out of a context in which intense individualism of authorship, as that prevailing in our present literary world, was unknown. Its acceptance as canon is evidence that it has been judged as *not* being unique to its authors. Certainly in Western civilization there have been enormous differences, varying with time and place, in the degree to which people have regarded the Bible as expressing specifiable individual minds. Yet there is no other single document that is comparable to it in expressing the collective being of Western civilization.

The Book of Job especially commends itself to our attention. It deals with suffering, the psychological suffering associated with the loss of children and property, and physical suffering in the form of boils. It arises from and directs our attention to both the crisis in life of man, the crisis that in some way must take place in the life of each individual who lives into adulthood, and a historical crisis in the Judeo-Christian tradition, the crisis associated with the transition from Judaism to Christianity.

The Book of Job also commends itself to our attention in the context of our previous discussion because of a particular insight I believe it contains: that there is an intrinsic relationship among separation-estrangement, physical disease, and the psychological condition associated with sacrifice. Earlier I reviewed a number of studies indicating a linkage between various forms of separation-estrangement and disease. The Book of Job is also significant in that it brings sacrifice, to which we were brought in considering pain, into focus.

Let us consider the manifest level of the Book of Job. It begins with a double disaster occurring to a seemingly righteous man. The protagonist of this drama, a victim of tragic occurrences, is visited by three friends, and, for most of the text, there is discussion relevant to the tragedies. The book, it seems, raises doubts about the justice of a God who would make a righteous man suffer. The rhetoric of the book presumes, as does so much of the Bible, the independent existence of a God, creator and overseer of the world, and raises the question how such a God might allow or even cause this suffering.

Let us bring to bear the modern discovery, basic to psychoanalytic thought, that the fantastic creations of man's mind arise out of the deepest parts of his psyche and that these fantastic creations are of man himself.

If there is a question for us of God's goodness or justice in the Book of Job, then we have to inquire about the nature of man who thus conceives of God. Indeed, the very ascription of evil to the divine, as such a hint exists in the Book of Job, is a hint to us of the nature of the psychological processes associated with suffering.

I have indicated that the canonical quality itself of the Bible is to be taken into account in using the Bible to understand the men whose collective mind it somehow expresses. We must take equal cognizance of the fact that there are special characteristics of the Book of Job affecting its canonical authenticity. The Book of Job stands, as it were, on the canonical margin. It is sometimes true that marginal instances may best help us to understand phenomena. The very characteristics of the Book of Job which provoke questions of its canonical authenticity are, I believe, significant for understanding the meaning of the book. I believe further that the Book of Job is distinguished both because it deals rather directly with the profoundest problems in the biblical mind and because its latent content is only thinly disguised. The former demands that it be regarded as part of the canon; the latter, that it be rejected. Allowing it to stay in the canon while it carries earmarks suggestive of canonical inauthenticity is a way of handling those problems.

The canonical marginality of the Book of Job is evident in the rough handling it received by the rabbis of the Talmud. They suggest that Job never existed; that he was not an Israelite;[2] that his name is a disguised

[2] A historical subscription in the Septuagint also indicates this. After 42:17 the Septuagint asserts that Job was a grandchild of Esau. Since Esau was the brother of Jacob (Israel), Job would then not be an Israelite.

form of the word meaning "enemy";[3] and that he and the other personages of the Book of Job were prophets for heathens rather than for Israel.[4] The latter suggests that the Book of Job might not properly belong in the Old Testament at all.

The book has characteristics that invite the reader to wonder about its authenticity. Theodore of Mopsuestia (d. 428) omitted it from his canon of the Bible, regarding it as a work of fiction. It consists of at least two radically different parts, one being in prose and the other in poetry. Because of this, scholars have maintained that there must have been at least two authors. The prose part, comprising the beginning and the end, chapters 1 and 2, and chapter 42:7–17, is regarded as having been composed by a considerably less skilled and experienced writer than the other. The long poetic part, which begins with 3:2, is manifestly the work of a talented and accomplished author.[5] The substantive problem presented by the text is never quite resolved. The book closes with a *deus ex machina* type of ending, all things set to rights, giving the tragedy a simple but very contrived "happy ending," as it were. And even here there are some peculiarities. Although the Book of Job closes with the rhetoric of a happy ending, Job dies with its final sentence. Death is, of course, usually associated with tragedy. Furthermore, simple replacements are provided for the children who were killed at the beginning of the book, as though this could compensate for the death of the others. Kallen has cogently argued that

[3] The transposition of the two middle characters of the Hebrew of Job's name yields "enemy." See footnote 11, p. 106.

[4] *The Talmud: Baba Bathra*, 15a ff., trans. M. Simon and I. W. Slotki (London: Soncino Press, 1935), pp. 73 ff.

[5] W. B. Stevenson, *The poem of Job* (London: Oxford University Press, 1947), p. 21.

the book is really quite marginal to the Jewish tradition, that it is a Hebraized version of a Greek tragedy after the style of Euripides, and that it reflects the crisis in Jewish history and thought when it was confronted by Greek civilization.[6] Kallen shows how by simple rearrangement of the lines the Book of Job may readily take on the appearance of an authentic Greek drama, demonstrating that it could thus have been an original form of the drama. It may be that the rabbis also sensed the to them odious Greek influence.

The book has been rather unimportant in Jewish history. As one reviewer of this history has put it, "All in all, it appears that Job has made a far greater impression upon the Christian than the Jewish group." Its reading among Jews, he maintains, has been with "solemnity, but inattention."[7] From the point of view of traditional Judaism there is considerable substance in the assertion by one scholar that "it is clear that Job's words were generally less in agreement with religious principles than were those of his three comforters."[8] The doubt which forms much of the substance of the book is somehow echoed in doubt concerning the canonical authenticity of the book.

The very artfulness of the Book of Job is also relevant. It has a self-consciously literary quality. It strongly urges the reader to look at it as a book. The poetic form of the central portion invites the reader to consider it a deliberate work of art rather than a narrative report of events. Indeed, certain lines in the book point to a literary awareness, as in "Oh that my words were

[6] H. M. Kallen, *The Book of Job as a Greek tragedy* (New York: Moffat, Yard & Co., 1918).

[7] I. J. Gerber, *The psychology of the suffering mind* (New York: Jonathan David Co., 1951), p. 35.

[8] Stevenson, *The poem of Job*, p. 22.

102

now written! oh that they were printed in a book!" (19:23), and, "Oh that one would hear me! behold, my desire is, that the Almighty would answer me, and that mine adversary had written a book" (31:35).

But what is a book? Among other things a book demands of the reader that he classify it as fiction or non-fiction, as fantasy or fact, as modern librarians characteristically do for us. The Book of Job seems somehow more fictional than perhaps any other book of the Bible. The ancients presumably did not draw the line between fact and fiction as firmly as we do, but the decision that the Book of Job should be part of the canon was undoubtedly informed by a decision that it should be regarded as non-fiction, as based on fact.

The hints of canonical inauthenticity, as well as the literary qualities which suggest that it is fiction, may be interpreted as serving psychologically to defend against the manifestation of the latent content of the book. They make it possible to reject the book should the latent content break through. The problem with which the text is grappling is so profound that the psychological defense of its possibly being outside of the canon or being fictional, combined with the characteristic strengthening of faith associated with doubt, have played their role in making it a significant expression of Western civilization. Fiction allows the reader to consider in detail the deepest psychological and existential questions without having to face the danger of a concrete threatening reality. In the entertainment of fiction, no matter what cognitive or affective or fantasied volitional activities one may engage in, there is always the defense that, after all, it is only fiction. Learning that the unbelievable is to be believed creates doubt. At the same time, overcoming doubt gives faith a tenacity which is otherwise unattainable. The psychological mechanism expressed by *credo quia absurdum est* against a background of doubt has long been associated with religious belief and is the reason why some religions have thrived on miracles. No one has ever thought about a reported miracle without at least a shadow of doubt crossing his mind. In overcoming that doubt, faith becomes a hard alloy.

Job, Abraham, and the Infanticidal Impulse

What then is the latent content in the Book of Job that led the biblical mind to defend against its manifestation? At this point we need to consider the infanticidal impulse, picking up a line of thought I have discussed elsewhere.[9] Freud's notion of the Oedipus complex certainly recognized the psychological significance of the identifications and conflicts in the father-son relationship. I believe, however, that Freud did not carry this sufficiently far to recognize that the Oedipus complex might itself be a reaction of the child to the infanticidal impulse in the father—Laius leaving Oedipus to die as a child—and a defensive response of the child against aggression. The infanticidal impulse in the male is associated, in Western civilization, with patrilineality and the assumption by the male of the responsibility of caring for the children. The infanticidal impulse is the reverse of this assumption of responsibility. Various regulations of traditional Judaism, such as the redemption of the first-born and the wearing of phylacteries, may be interpreted as efforts to counteract the infanticidal impulse. Christianity may also be interpreted

[9] D. Bakan, *The duality of human existence: an essay on psychology and religion* (Chicago: Rand McNally, 1966), pp. 205 ff.

as an effort to counteract this infanticidal impulse, having arisen against a background in which the then classical Jewish modes of dealing with this impulse were faltering, as witness especially the holocaust of infant slaughter under Herod from which Jesus was saved. Christianity provided new devices for handling the impulse, especially in the sacrifice of the Mass.

That the Book of Job opens with the death of Job's children, and that the death of the children is a critical part of Job's tragedy and fate, suggests the same problem, the management of the infanticidal impulse. The book may therefore provide the appearance of fictionality and canonical inauthenticity in order to defend against this latent content. It is thus rendered ostensibly as a "story," which ought perhaps not to have been made part of the canon.

The Book of Job is continuous with the story of Abraham; and one might well assume that the story of Job is highly conditioned by the story of Abraham. Abraham is the major figure in the Old Testament representing the shift of the adult male into a position of accepting biological bondage of the father to the child. The story of Abraham's move to sacrifice Isaac is indicative of the infanticidal impulse. The fact that Abraham's arm is restrained is indicative of the effectiveness of the contra-infanticidal tendencies.

The relationship of the Job story to the story of Abraham was evidently quite taken for granted by the rabbis of the Talmud. In their commentary on the opening to the Book of Job they ascribe the following words to Satan: "Sovereign of the Universe, I have traversed the whole world and found none so faithful as thy servant Abraham."[10]

[10] *The Talmud: Baba Bathra*, pp. 76–77.

Job and Abraham are presented to the reader principally as fathers. Both have relationships with God in which the major concern is with offspring. Their names are similar. Abraham's names in the Old Testament are first AVRM (Abram) and then AVRHM (Abraham), with AV meaning father. Job's name is AYOV, with the first and last letters also being AV.[11] As Abraham is visited by three men (Gen. 18), so is Job. (Three men also appear at the birth of the infant Jesus.) As Abraham is described as righteous, so is Job. As God concocted a test of Abraham entailing the death of his offspring, so does he do with Job. As Abraham is described as dying in great age, so is Job (Gen. 25:8; Job 42:17).

But the Book of Job differs dramatically from the story of Abraham in the following respect: whereas, in the story of Abraham the child is not killed, in the Book of Job the children are killed. Although in both instances there is a test of righteousness involved, the test for Abraham is whether he would kill Isaac; but the test for Job is his response to the killing of his children.

The story of the children's being killed is a fantasy in the biblical mind of their being killed. And a fantasy of their being killed suggests a wish that they be killed. The Book of Job begins with God and Satan involved in a plot to kill Job's children. The attribution of the infanticidal activity to God and Satan is a thin disguise. In spite of the fact that the killing of the children is attributed to these supernatural beings, the fact is that

[11] Such a liberty of suggestion as I am taking here is not at all inconsistent with similar liberties with letters, words, and names in the Jewish tradition. There is, for example, a similar use of such a device in the Talmud in transposing AYOV (Job) to AOYV (enemy) (*The Talmud: Baba Bathra*, p. 81). It would not have been at all inconsistent with the Jewish tradition to have signaled a relationship between Job and Abraham in this manner.

the Book of Job was written by men and constitutes
their fantasy.

Let us again consider the possibility that the fictional
quality of the Book of Job is a defense against making
manifest that which it contains latently. As I have already indicated, the first two chapters of the Book of
Job and the last differ radically from the remainder. Indeed, modern translations, including the Revised Version of the English Bible of 1611, use different type
styles for them.[12] This stylistic feature seems to convey
to the reader that the central poetic portion is the substantive part of the book and that the substantially
shorter beginning and the end are merely rhetorically
introductory and concluding material. Many critics, in
point of fact, responded to the Book of Job by directing
their attention principally to the central poetic portion
and paying little or no attention to the beginning and
the end. If there is an infanticidal theme in the Book of
Job, however, it is far more evident in the beginning and
the end than in the central longer poetic part. The radically different and more insistent style of that much
larger portion of the book tends thus to obscure the infanticidal theme, which is closer to being manifest in
the shorter prose part.

Even within the central poetic portion, however,
there is at least one indication of the infanticidal impulse, and this too is made to appear extraneous to the
text. The "Poem of the Ostrich" describes how the
ostrich jeopardizes her eggs:

> Gavest thou the goodly wings unto the peacocks?
> or wings and feathers unto the ostrich?
> Which leaveth her eggs in the earth, and warmeth
> them in dust,

[12] Stevenson, *The poem of Job*, p. 21.

And forgetteth that the foot may crush them, or
that the wild beast may break them.

She is hardened against her young ones, as
though they were not hers: her labor is in vain
without fear;

Because God hath deprived her of wisdom,
neither hath he imparted to her understanding.

What time she lifteth up herself on high, she
scorneth the horse and his rider.   [Job 39:13–18]

Stevenson, in his textual analysis of the Book of Job,
points out that the "Poem of the Ostrich" is not only
substantively different from the context but is also different in poetic form. It consists of a six-line stanza,
whereas the other stanzas in the text are of either four
or eight lines.[13] He is, furthermore, of the opinion that
the "Poem of the Ostrich" is best kept apart from the
rest of the poem. It is impossible to exclude it from the
Book of Job. It is simply there. But this critic's response means that the reader must recognize that there
are features of this particular poem which suggest the
possibility that it *might* be considered apart from the
rest. It is particularly interesting that this very stanza,
poetically different from its context, should be one in
which the infanticidal impulse is so clearly depicted; in
which it is indicated that God creates infanticidal
creatures.

It is rather interesting that the rabbis of the Talmud
also gave an infanticidal interpretation to a line very
close, in the same chapter, as the "Poem of the Ostrich."
This is the line: "Knowest thou the time when the wild
goats of the rock bring forth?" (39:1). The interpretation of this line is: "This wild goat is heartless toward
her young. When she crouches for delivery, she goes up

[13] *Ibid.*, pp. 23–24.

to the top of a mountain so that the young shall fall down and be killed, and I prepare an eagle to catch it in his wings and set it before her, and if he were one second too soon or too late it would be killed."[14] Thus the Talmud could attribute an infanticidal interpretation to a line even more obscure than the "Poem of the Ostrich."

Aside from such considerations suggesting an infanticidal theme latently contained in the Book of Job, the book also ascribes to Job a certain coldness toward his children. Job's ten children are counted with the number of his sheep, camels, oxen, and she-asses, as though they too were livestock and property. The loss of the children is recited among the losses of the livestock. At the end of the story, when all things appear to be rectified, he is granted children and livestock together, as though dead children were simply replaceable by live ones as were animals. Furthermore, Job does not mourn for *them*. His distress is hardly mourning in the sense of being possessed with the tragedy of *their* death. His distress, quite the contrary, is over *his* losses and the anguish of his body. Nowhere in the text is there any indication that he bewails the fate of his dead children. Indeed, upon learning of the loss of his livestock and children he comments: "Naked came I out of my mother's womb, and naked shall I return thither: the Lord gave, and the Lord hath taken away; blessed be the name of the Lord" (1:21). His first comment to his friends is equally egocentric: "Let the day perish wherein I was born, and the night in which it was said, There is a man child conceived" (3:3).

The text indicates that it was the custom of Job's children to engage in feasts together, but that Job him-

---

[14] *The Talmud: Baba Bathra*, p. 81.

self was not among them. Job is said to have occupied himself differently:

> And it was so, when the days of their feasting were gone about, that Job sent and sanctified them, and rose up early in the morning, and offered burnt offerings according to the number of them all: for Job said, It may be that my sons have sinned, and cursed God in their hearts. Thus did Job continually [1:5].

We have here the suggestion of Job's alienation from his children in not being companion to their drinking and feasting, his clearly indicated suspicion of them, and his clearly indicated sacrifice on their behalf. I take it that, as in the story of Abraham, Job's sacrifices are central to our understanding of the Book of Job.

The Voices of the Victims

Let us assume that behind the biblical text there is a latent myth that the victims of infanticidal acts, the slain children, are "Sons of God." Thus, if the Book of Job is critically based on a latent infanticidal impulse, and if it constitutes an effort to come to terms with the impulse, it is appropriate that the story should begin with a gathering of the "Sons of God," come seeking justice. "Now there was a day when the sons of God came to present themselves before the Lord, and Satan came also among them" (Job 1:6). Satan, as I have suggested elsewhere, should be thought of as among "whatsoever openeth the womb" (Exod. 13:2) and as victim.[15]

There is a sequence of two challenges of Job at Satan's

[15] Bakan, *Duality of human existence*, p. 59.

instigation. Job first loses his livestock and children. Since Job, evidently, does not sin as a result of this, Satan makes the second challenge: "Skin for skin, yea, all that a man hath will he give for his life. But put forth thine hand now, and touch his bone and his flesh, and he will curse thee to thy face" (2:4–5). If we interpret Satan to be himself one of the victimized, and spokesman for all of them, he is, in effect, charging that certainly justice for the crime of infanticide has not been done by depriving Job of his livestock and especially his children; and justice remains to be done by injuring Job's body directly.

Thus, one way of interpreting the Book of Job is as a story of the "Sons of God" coming back to haunt the child-killer or, at least, as an expression of the state of mind haunted by that complex in which the infanticidal impulse is the nucleus. Job's speeches just before the appearance of Elihu, whom I shall discuss momentarily, contain protestations of how well he took care of the young and the needy (30, 31). It is immediately following these speeches that Elihu, the youth and possible victim, is introduced, speaking angrily in reply to Job's self-justifications (32:2).

At this point it is worth our while to turn slightly from the direct consideration of the Book of Job to a consideration of the New Testament, of which the Book of Job is certainly a harbinger. At the Last Supper, as this is described in John, after Jesus has identified Judas and instructed him, "That thou doest, do quickly" (13:27), he says, "Little children, yet a little while I am with you" (13:33), suggesting that soon Jesus too would be among the other victims of the infanticidal impulse, among the other "Sons of God." Jesus, I believe, understood himself to be the victim of the infanticidal impulse. He was an opener of the womb and so belonged

111

to God. I suggest that the term "Son of God" has as one of its functions removal of the sense of guilt engendered by the infanticidal impulse.

The appearance of Elihu in the Book of Job constitutes a further literary peculiarity. His appearance is extraneous to the manifest structure of the book. Job, it would seem, has been the victim of tragedy and three friends properly come to console him. The dialogue goes on among Job and his three friends. And then, quite out of nowhere, the speech of Elihu appears. In some respects the literary device is similar to the one pointed out in connection with the "Poem of the Ostrich," in which material is presented that allows and even invites itself to be put apart from the rest of the text. Elihu, too, should be thought of as a possible target of the infanticidal impulse; he is, in this respect, a transitional figure between Isaac and Jesus, between Isaac, who was spared, and Jesus, who was not. Indeed, there is a traditional view that Elihu really is Isaac.[16] The text takes great pains to have the reader understand that Elihu is young. Although there is no prior mention of him, his earlier presence is taken for granted in the text, since his remarks indicate that he has been listening to what has been said by the others. He challenges the elders, contending that they are not always wise or understanding, in much the same way that Jesus does when he proclaims that that which is hidden from the wise and the prudent is revealed to the babes (Matt. 11:25; Luke 10:21). I have earlier suggested that what Jesus was referring to was the existence of the infanticidal impulse in adults.[17]

[16] L. Ginzberg, *The legends of the Jews,* trans. Henrietta Szold (Philadelphia: Jewish Publication Society, 1961), 1: 326. Based on Yerushalmi Sotah 5, 20d.

[17] Bakan, *Duality of human existence,* pp. 222 ff.

Elihu's position on the issue differs dramatically from the positions of the three friends, Eliphaz, Bildad, and Zophar. They tend to conceive of the relationship between man and God as rational, even contractual, with God being the dispenser of the rewards and punishments. It is from this perspective that they seek somehow to find reason for Job's suffering. Elihu's comments, however, are not legalistic in this sense but are rather like those of a child who has no alternative but to trust— the voice of the child who is in the hands of the father. The father is his creator: "The Spirit of God hath made me, and the breath of the Almighty hath given me life" (33:4). God "giveth not account of any of his matters" (33:13). "Touching the Almighty, we cannot find him out: he is excellent in power, and in judgment, and in plenty of justice: he will not afflict" (37:23).

A Son, Not a Father

Psychologically the Book of Job may be regarded as expressing a transition from the state of mind of father to the state of mind of son, the change coming about as a defense against the guilt associated with the infanticidal impulse. This change is important for understanding the emergence of Christianity. In it the many varieties of suffering to which the human being is subject are reinterpreted in the model of a child as victim of the father. The infanticidal impulse is apparently got rid of by projecting it. Guilt is reduced because one appears to one's self as the victim rather than as the infanticidal father. At the same time, however, it conceptualizes suffering and especially death as being under the will, albeit someone else's will, and thus allows the logical possibility of immortality as a function of will. If death comes only at the will of God, and if God could be persuaded to decide in one's favor, then might one live forever. If there is any guilt associated with audaciously willing to live forever, this guilt is removed by ascribing it to God. It is of note that nowhere in the whole of the Book of Job is there even a suggestion that Job's suffering might have natural causes independent of God's will. There is only one cause for all of Job's suffering, the will of God. The book is an attempt to take on the voice of trust of the child in his father, who is conceived of as all-powerful, and who is in the first instance the very creator of being.

These considerations help us to appreciate the important difference between Job and Abraham. Abraham contracted with God to care for his children after he was gone. Job, in contrast, having psychologically engaged in infanticide, as it were, strains to identify himself with the victim, subject to injury only by God. This identification is the fusion of the one who kills with the one who is killed, which Freud conceptualized as the internalizing of the father into the psyche as the superego. Our earlier discussion indicated this mechanism as a major factor in human suffering.

If death is only through the will of a God who can grant eternal life, and he spares not even one, then one who may be caught in the whirlpool of this construction is brought to the point of reproaching God. Indeed one piece of liturgy which, I believe, is illuminated by interpreting it as a reproach, is the Kaddish said by Jewish mourners. It is little more than praise of God. But it appears to have the implicit meaning, in addition, that if God is so great, why has he allowed or caused this? Job's initial reaction, that "the Lord gave, and the Lord hath taken away; blessed be the name of the Lord" (1:21) may also be interpreted as the victim justifying the infanticidal act of the father. It is the father who made being in the first place, and therefore it is his right to undo it. But justification is always built on reproach, explicit or implicit. If this first response is only a veiled reproach, the second response is less veiled: "Let the day perish wherein I was born, and the night in which it was said, There is a man child conceived" (3:3). This is the Freudian Oedipus complex reproach, the reproach against the father for having engaged in the act which led to one's creation. It is a reproach against the father for having created him if he was to kill him later; a reproach against the sexuality of the father out of which the child was conceived; and a reproach against one's self insofar as one is thus the lustful and infanticidal father. The Christian idea of the virgin birth, succeeding as it does the story of Job, carries the reproach even further; for it even denies the relationship to the father, and denies him his procreative role. Against a background of a culture engaged in a struggle to maintain the dominance of the patrilineal idea, a culture struggling to make men identify with their children as their "seed," the idea of the virgin birth also defends against the guilt of the father for killing the child; for in the major infanticide in history the victim is said to have had no human biological father. Paradoxically, of course, the New Testament still endows Jesus with a completely patrilineal genealogy (Matt. 1:1–17). We need thus to recognize that Job's denunciation of his own conception is a reproach against the father for his infanticidal tendencies; and that one psychological solution to the problem of the guilt of infanticide is to move from the role of the father to the role of son. Job's answer to tragedy is to announce that he is to be understood as a child, as a son and not as a father. In effect, Job, psychologically the slayer of children, is depicted

115

as attempting to hide among the children, adding his voice to the children's chorus. Yet in so doing, living or dying becomes a prerogative of will, even if it has to be God's will.

Sacrifice as Righteousness

The Book of Job explicitly indicates that Job is righteous, but, at the same time, it contains allusions suggesting that he is involved in the deepest of sins. How can one be both simultaneously? I suggest that by answering this riddle we may understand suffering better; and that, furthermore, we can answer this riddle by considering that one activity, sacrifice, which, according to the text, Job is said to have engaged in with great conscientiousness.

There is a clue in a statement attributed to Job's wife in the text: "Dost thou still retain thine integrity? curse God, and die" (2:9). In order to appreciate its significance we must return to the Hebrew. The word translated as "curse" is not curse at all, but "bless." The context is such, however, that the translator is quite correct in interpreting "bless" as a euphemism for "curse." The suggestion is very strong that "bless" and "curse" are deeply intertwined, that they are, in some sense, one. The principal act of righteousness is sacrifice. It is precisely in sacrifice that "bless" and "curse" coalesce. If this is how Job expresses his righteousness, it is both "bless" and "curse."

Consider again the story of Abraham and Isaac, the paradigmatic sacrifice tale. That story is indicative of profound ambivalence. On the one hand, there is Abraham's wish for many children and for God to provide them with land and eternal protection. On the other hand, there is the wish to kill Isaac, although the latter wish is projected onto God also, appearing as God's command to Abraham. When a human being inflicts pain upon another human being, he characteristically believes that he does so out of necessity. In the case of Abraham it is out of obedience to God. But one can reasonably ask about the locus of the necessity. A common psychodynamic mechanism is to convert desire so that it appears as external necessity. It is thus an open question in each instance whether what appears to be external necessity really is that, or is simply a façade concealing some internal pressure. The externalization of necessity is often buttressed by both an ultra-mythicism and an ultra-realism. Both were present, for example, in the great holocaust of naziism, with the revival of German historical myths, on the one hand, and the complete banality—to borrow Hannah Arendt's term for it—and excessive realism of orderliness, obedience, bureaucracy, files, schedules, supplies, etc., of Eichmann, on the other. Although ultra-mythicism and ultra-realism appear to be poles apart, they are identical in that in both there is the externalization of necessity. There is only a superficial contrast between them.

The appearance of the ram at the last moment indicates the possibility of substituting an animal for Abraham's son. Psychologically, however, the sacrifice of an animal is then also symbolic of killing the son. Since if A is a substitute for B, then A is also symbolic of B, killing an animal instead of a son is a symbolic way of killing the son. In the story of Abraham, the substitution of an animal appears to resolve the conflict. The ram is killed, and Isaac is spared.

In contrast to the Abraham and Isaac story, the Book of Job is indicative of a state of mind for which the use of animals as a way of appeasing the infanticidal im-

117

pulse has lost its effectiveness. By the time the Book of Job was composed, the strong distinction between animals and children had become considerably blurred in the biblical mind. All of Job's sacrificing of animals has been to no avail. He is said to have lost animals and children simultaneously. If the distinction between children and animals is drawn either very sharply, or if the distinction is very blurred, then the sacrifice of animals gives little satisfaction to the infanticidal impulse. If it is the former, the distinction between child and animal makes it impossible to feel that the child is being killed in the killing of the animal. If it is the latter, then one moves to killing the children with the same impunity as one kills animals. It is this second situation that we encounter in the Book of Job.

Wherein, then, lies Job's righteousness? In the biblical mind righteousness consists in part in making sacrifices; and this Job has clearly done. It is not only in action that righteousness consists, however, but also in a certain condition of mind. Righteousness would also consist in being able to maintain a balanced distinction between children and animals so that, as in the case of the righteous Abraham, a ram could substitute for Isaac. The question of the Book of Job really is, as indeed the rabbis of the Talmud took it to be, whether Job was as righteous as Abraham. For in the Book of Job it is not at all clear. Job is said to have sacrificed, but the children died. Abraham sacrificed but Isaac lived on that account. Genuine righteousness should at least consist in being able to maintain a piety that does its psychological work. In the Book of Job the problem is whether piety does the work it is supposed to do. The book rather bespeaks a state of mind in which the distinction between children and animals was not maintained, a state of mind going toward an acted-out infanticidal

118

impulse. Had the state of the biblical mind been such as to win a sense of satisfaction for the infanticidal impulse from the sacrifice of animals, it is unlikely that the Book of Job would have been composed or written down.

The child who may be killed by the father is ambiguously both someone else and the father himself. The substitution of familial immortality for individual immortality is among the important psychological efforts represented in the Old Testament. There is hardly a page in the Bible on which it is not asserted in one way or another that the male can have children. There is an overlay of one conflict upon another in the biblical mind, for which sacrifice was such a significant act. There is an initial conflict between individual survival and survival through one's offspring. If one opts for individual survival rather than survival through one's offspring, another conflict arises. Shall one survive by being an adult and killing the child or by being a child to the "father," deferring to him so that he will not kill one as the "child"? Taking the child's role spares one from the temptations of infanticide. Taking the child's role also opens up the possibility of endless life, since the termination of life has been converted into something dependent only on the sufferance of the "father." If he can be appeased, one might live forever. But taking the role of the child means surrendering sexuality, reproduction, and one's own fatherhood—which, indeed, developed into an ideal of Christianity—and thus not having available the possibility of immortality through one's offspring. One is left only with personal immortality; and personal mortality is inexorable.

The conflicts posed by the Abraham and Isaac story are between the two ways of surviving as an individual: between killing the child so that one will survive one's self and infantile deference to the father so that one will not be killed by him. Whichever of these means is taken would remove the possibility of survival through one's offspring. In the Abraham and Isaac story the way out of the conflict was symbolic: an animal was sacrificed instead of a child. By sacrificing an animal one does not kill the child and is therefore not "cut off" by the act. One also defers to the "father" by sacrificing to him and thus preventing him from killing one, thereby opening the possibility of personal immortality. And one satisfies the infanticidal impulse at least symbolically.

In contrast, Job, for all his sacrificing, is "cut off," at least until the restoration at the end of the book. The biblical expression "cut off" means to be killed, to be socially ostracized, and, in particular, to be childless. It might be pointed out parenthetically that Freud's use of the notion of "castration" as a concretization of the most drastic punishment was perhaps conditioned by the biblical tradition, in that literal castration involves simultaneously a threat to the life of the individual, the consequent impossibility of having intercourse (and thus of entering into that which Freud took to be paradigmatic of all intimate interpersonal—social—relations), and the impossibility of having children.

Sacrifice and Individual Survival

The fact that animals also constituted a major source of food supply serves to confound the meaning of sacrifice. The discussion thus far suggests that the ritual of sacrifice entailed two different psychological substitutions. First, the one for whose sake the sacrifice is made has been shifted from the father to God, essentially ascribing to God the infanticidal impulse of the father. Second, the victim of the sacrifice has been shifted from child to animal. We can deepen our understanding of the matter by observing the significance of the issue of the food supply.

Although the text indicates that Job is a wealthy man in terms of his possession of animals, giving their precise number and describing him as "the greatest of all the men of the east" by virtue of his "substance" (1:3), there is also a hint that the food supply is an issue when we compare the beginning and the end of the Book of Job. At the beginning of the book the text indicates that the brothers undertook the responsibility for feeding their sisters: "And his sons went and feasted in their houses, every one his day; and sent and called for their three sisters to eat and to drink with them" (1:4). At the end of the book, when Job's wealth is doubly restored to him, the text indicates that Job gave to the replaced daughters "inheritance among their brethren" (42:15), as though the authors wished to make sure that readers would understand that Job is finally providing for his daughters. The Septuagint version of the Book of Job is much more explicit about poverty having been an issue. It includes words from Job's wife in which she speaks of herself as "wandering about, or working for wages, from place to place and from house to house, wishing for the setting of the sun, that I may rest from the labours and sorrows I endure" (2:9).

We may presume that the biblical mind had learned one of the most primitive forms of "investment," to allow children to grow up as a provision against starvation in the future, analogous to allowing an animal to mature and to breed instead of eating it. Such an "investment policy" required, however, that the young be indoctrinated with a sense of responsibility for providing for those who had spared them in their childhood. Young persons rendering meat to the old is a ubiquitous theme

121

in the Bible. It may be seen in the story of Cain and Abel, where the text indicates that "the Lord had respect unto Abel and to his offering" of meat (Gen. 4:4), "but unto Cain and to his offering [of the fruit of the ground] he had not respect" (Gen. 4:5). There is the similar story of the demand by Isaac in his role as father for "savoury meat, such as I love" (Gen. 27:4) before giving the blessing. Indeed, obligation in the Bible is often exactly that of rendering meat offerings and other food to God. If the meat served is meat of animals, and it is in abundance, the conflict between the temptation of killing children and deference is hardly aroused. When there is shortage, however, the conflict between getting rid of children to conserve food and allowing them to grow up so that they can then supply food to their elders is aroused. The biblical references to child sacrifice are numerous, and one might suspect that, at times, when conditions were dire, a cannibalistic impulse was aroused in the biblical mind. That this is at least a possibility is indicated by the story told in 2 Kings, in which two women arranged that on one day they would eat the child of one and on another they would eat the child of the other. One of them bitterly complains over being betrayed: "So we boiled my son, and did eat him: and I said unto her on the next day, Give thy son, that we may eat him: and she hath hid her son" (6:29).

Thus, under conditions of shortage the biblical mind is brought to sin, brought to the killing of the children. If righteousness consists, in any part, in keeping the father supplied, and there is a shortage of food, and it is in some sense believed that the shortage is itself due to inadequate deference to the "father," the impulse to kill the child—seemingly as an act of righteousness—is aroused. Thus, paradoxically, the major sin in the first place, killing the children, becomes what appears to be an act of righteousness, although, in the last analysis, killing the child is deference of the individual to his personal survival.

This deep paradox of the Judeo-Christian tradition, the convergence of the ultimate of righteousness and the ultimate of sin, is the basic theme of the Book of Job, even on the manifest level. Job's bitterness is the bitterness of confronting this paradox. The paradox is rooted in the fact that each generation is a transition between generations, and each would itself be immortal. Job comes to terms with this by allowing that there is a God, who is different from himself, and that the ways of this God are incomprehensible to man. The attribution of incomprehensibility to God, which is a major theological contribution of the Book of Job, allows the possibility that the paradox has a resolution, albeit unknown to man.

We may interpret the Book of Job as indicating that sacrifice is ultimately unsatisfactory as a psychological mechanism. Job's sacrificing is the beginning and hardly the end of his difficulties. In seeming righteousness, the biblical mind in the Book of Job fulfills the wish to kill the children and comes to the realization that in the ultimate act of righteousness one is "cut off."

It has been recognized in the psychoanalytic literature that, although an unfulfilled wish may be involved in creating a neurotic condition, the resolution of the neurotic condition does not inhere in the satisfaction of the wish. We see this, for example, in the story of Oedipus and in Freud's treatment of the Oedipus complex. Freud identified what he took as one of the deepest wishes, that of having sexual relations with one's mother, in the story of Oedipus. Yet the fulfillment of the wish hardly brought happiness to Oedipus. Indeed, the fulfillment is the major condition of the tragedy. Similarly, the fantastic satisfaction of the wish does not result in happiness or fulfillment but is the nucleus of tragedy in the Book of Job. The sacrifice of animals failed either to appease the father or to satisfy the infanticidal wish in the biblical mind.

In the Book of Job that mind has moved to the fantasy of engaging in the sacrifice of the children. But this fails; for then one is "cut off" and there is no possible comfort in the idea that one may be immortal through one's offspring. They are dead.

The Sacrifice of Self and Mortality

The biblical mind is thus brought to entertain the sacrifice of one's self. As the story has it, Satan is not satisfied that Job's children or his animals are dead. He must suffer disease. Only disease can satisfy the psychological logic of the biblical mind. Here we return to a theme we have dealt with before, how with respect to destructive impulses the psyche has difficulty in maintaining the distinction between that which is self and that which is other, so that often the same destructive impulses may work at once toward the injury of one's self and the injury of others.

A confounding of self and other is present from the beginning in sacrifice. One gives up what one loves— "giving up" being ambiguously intransitive and transitive. On the one hand, sacrifice is transitive, entailing the killing of someone else. On the other hand, sacrifice is intransitive, entailing surrender of an important part of one's self for the "redemption" of the remainder. It is exactly the same mechanism that I identified in the discussion of pain, where a part of the body becomes "it" in preparation for its sacrifice. To engage in sacrifice is

124

to kill another organism; yet that other organism's loss of life constitutes a loss to the person who is sacrificing.

Sacrifice is a manifestation of telic decentralization. A part of the self is made into an "it" for the seeming preservation of the remainder. But the act of sacrifice is already part of the process that leads to death. The psychological function of sacrifice, insofar as it has value, rests on a confounding which in and of itself constitutes the basis for the ultimate death of the organism. Unless that which is sacrificed is in some sense one's self, it cannot work, and hence the double challenge of Satan in the Book of Job. Insofar as that which is sacrificed is one's self, the realization must come quickly that one is being evasive in sacrificing the other and that, if one is to sacrifice at all, one should sacrifice one's self directly. The authors of the Book of Job in some sense appreciated what our more modern considerations and data reveal. The tragedy of Job at once involved the loss of his children and disease.

The profoundest complaint that man can make to his creator is that, having made him, he made him mortal. An essential feature of man's condition is expressed metaphorically in the Genesis story, in which there are two trees: man ate only of one of them and was cast forth from the Garden of Eden to prevent him from eating of the Tree of Life and living forever (Gen. 3:22). Having eaten of the first tree, he is capable of wisdom, understanding, and knowledge, the latter connoting and including generativity. But the fact of the matter is that individual man is mortal, and there is no way in which to stop the inexorable movement toward the death of the individual organism. Sacrifice might support an illusory hope of immortality, but it is only an illusion. Even the amputee whose life is saved by the sacrifice of his limb will eventually die. At some point the truth

125

comes through that nothing one can do will make one's individual being immortal. For all of Job's sacrificing he must die. An immortal father-God who *might* spare man is a hollow fantasy, and to believe it costs man his maturity.

Contemplating the Book of Job helps us to appreciate one of the major defects of the Judeo-Christian tradition, the tendency to subsume death under punishment, to leave out the possibility of death which is not punishment. To conceive of death as resulting only from lack of virtue is essentially to adopt a view of death characteristic of the thought of a child, for whom neglect by or hostility from adults is the most likely cause of death. So conceiving of death perverts the fact that death is inevitable in time and will occur whether the life lived has been virtuous or not. Virtue might be associated with longevity, but it does not provide immortality.

In the Book of Job the cause of disease is attributed basically to God. But the fact remains that all human beings must eventually become diseased of something and die. Much of the discussion that Job has with his friends assumes that God causes death in each instance. But Job, at times, appears wiser than his three friends. For to Job the authors attribute the recognition that just to be born entails a sentence of death (14:1 ff.). In the Book of Job there is a harbinger of the notion of "original sin," the sin in being born—that being born is the sin which is "punished" by the death to ensue in a finite number of days. "Man that is born of a woman is of few days" (14:1), for "Who can bring a clean thing out of an unclean? Not one" (14:4). Not until the biblical mind could accept a man born of an immaculate woman could it imagine one who would be quite immortal. Immaculate conception is a prerequisite for immortality. Without the one there could not be the other.

126

Man's death is in his nature, but not necessarily in his will. To "long for death" (3:21) is to assert the role of will even in connection with the inevitable death. The Judeo-Christian tradition has for centuries properly recognized the pride and sin associated with suicide. To "long for death," and to act on this longing, is to arrogate to one's own will what has been imposed on everyone for the "original sin" of having been born; and it is not proper to pre-empt the role of the executioner. If the act of sacrifice is, as I have indicated, an act of self-injury, it is equally an act of audacity. To kill is always to pre-empt the natural death of any organism, which is inevitable in any circumstances. It puts death under the control of the will, giving the illusion that otherwise there is immortality. Christianity is based on the recognition of the audacity associated with sacrifice. It makes the major sacrificial act of history one of God himself. The sacrifice was "begotten" of God; and it was a sacrifice "without blemish," a condition the Old Testament so often indicates is preferred by God for sacrifice.

The Book of Job seeks to refute the thesis that virtue and reward, vice and punishment, are necessarily associated. The ultimate refutation of this thesis in the biblical sequence is the story of Jesus, in which one who is eminently virtuous, even to the point of having been born without original sin, still suffers. The Book of Job is a step in this refutation because in it the seemingly righteous man is made to suffer precisely as a test of his righteousness. Job's quarrel with his friends is about their assumption that suffering follows sin and that the amount of suffering is regulated by the amount of sin, which Job rejects. For Job knows full well that his righteousness, or any righteousness, does not give immortality. He asserts that the association is null, and he comes to recognize the deep sinfulness of believing that there is a separate God who rewards virtue and punishes vice. For if such were the case one could work toward one's immortality by wilfully being righteous, which in itself would be an attempt to disobey God's wish that man not eat of the Tree of Life. In short, Job knows that it is sinful to believe that God rewards the righteous with immortality; he knows it is not true; he knows that death is inexorable.

There are two major points in life which are beyond the scope of the individual will. One is conception; the other is death. Between these, but not including them, the will of the individual has its proper sphere. To fancy one's self one's own creator, or to place death within the power of the will, are the real sins of mankind. This Job understands. And this, I believe, Freud understood when he stressed the fantasy of presence and witness to the primal scene, on the one hand, and the death instinct, on the other.

At the end of the Book of Job, God is presented as manifesting anger against Job's three friends, commanding them to "offer up for yourselves a burnt offering" (42:8). For them, who still believe in the relationship of virtue and vice to reward and punishment and who have not quite appreciated the fact that death is inexorable in spite of all, sacrifice is still an appropriate activity. But for Job the mechanism is no longer appropriate. He rather will have his children, will provide for them, and will sacrifice no more on behalf of them. After a long life he will die, comfortable in having eaten of the first tree, but no longer lusting after the second.

Index

Index

Index